AF598380

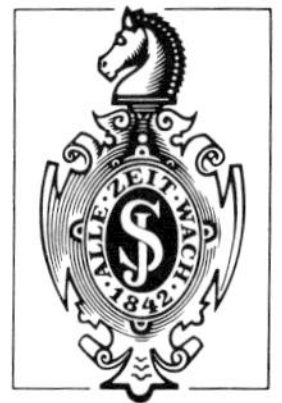

Fractures with Soft Tissue Injuries

Edited by
H. Tscherne and L. Gotzen

With 107 Figures

Springer-Verlag
Berlin Heidelberg New York Tokyo 1984

Prof. Dr. Harald Tscherne
Medizinische Hochschule, Unfallchirurgische Klinik
Postfach 610180, D-3000 Hannover 61

Prof. Dr. Leo Gotzen
Medizinische Hochschule, Unfallchirurgische Klinik
Postfach 610180, D-3000 Hannover 61

Translator: Terry C. Telger, 3054 Vaughan Avenue, Marina, CA 93933/USA

Title of the original German edition: *Fraktur und Weichteilschaden*

ISBN 3-540-12095-5 / 0-387-12095-5

ISBN 3-540-13082-9 Springer-Verlag Berlin Heidelberg New York Tokyo
ISBN 0-387-13082-9 Springer-Verlag New York Heidelberg Berlin Tokyo

Printing and binding: Beltz Offsetdruck, 6944 Hemsbach/Bergstr.
2124/3140-543210

Preface

Progress in medical science, and the deeping of physician experience in general, make continuing education a fundamental obligation on the part of the practicing physician. Besides academies of advanced medical training, we feel that medical schools and universities offer a particularly good setting for continuing medical education.

When the Hannover Medical School established West Germany's first Department of Trauma Surgery in 1970, we committed ourselves to this goal and instituted the Hannover Trauma Seminars as a regional forum for continuing physician education. Made up almost entirely of our colleagues at the Trauma Surgery Clinic, the basic goal of the seminars is to review new discoveries and techniques in the field of traumatology and assess their practical relevance to the physician who treats trauma victims. In addition to research, the experience of the Hannover School of Trauma Surgery form an important basis for seminar activities.

The first Trauma Seminar was held on February 2, 1972. Initially, copies of the proceedings were simply distributed to all interested participants. But as attendance grew and demand for the proceedings increased, it became necessary to seek a broader form of publication. Henceforth, the Hannover Trauma Seminars will be published as part of the *Topics in Traumatology* series. For this we are grateful to Springer Verlag and to series editors Jörg Rehn and Leonhard Schweiberer.

The current issue deals with fractures and associated soft tissue injuries. These common and often severe lesions are seen in a large percentage of multiple trauma patients, and they can be quite troublesome in terms of management. A thorough understanding of indications and therapy is needed in order to avoid infection and achieve a good end result.

The many problems posed by this type of injury are addressed in 11 papers, each of which supplements the others in points emphasized, yet is distinct in terms of this content. Clinical aspects are preceeded by a discussion of the pathophysiology of soft tissue trauma. This forms the basis for a new, clinically-oriented classification system which takes special account of closed fractures with soft tissue injury.

The general management of open fractures is explained, drawing upon techniques that have been successfully practiced at our center. The handling of open fractures at the accident scene and in the hospital, diagnostic procedures, preparations for surgery, and operative treatment are discussed in some detail. The special problems of closed fractures with soft tissue injury are addressed in a separate paper.

Much space has been devoted to the tibial region on account of its peculiar anatomy, the prevalence of tibial injuries, and the frequent severity of the trauma. The indications for operative fixation are outlined, and procedural details are given for various types and localizations of osseous and soft tissue injury.

The compartment syndrome is one of the most frequent and severe complications of fractures with soft tissue injury, yet its importance has not been fully appreciated in clinical practice. A separate paper is devoted to the etiology, pathophysiology, diagnosis and treatment of this condition so that the serious consequences of its neglect or delayed recognition may be avoided.

Sound postoperative management is an integral part of total patient care. Early complications are frequent and require prompt, judicious intervention. The successful treatment of fractures with soft tissue injury depends largely on the nature and extent of the damage to soft tissue structures. Isolated bone fragments, even if securely fixed, will eventually succomb to necrosis and predispose to infection. In this situation, plastic procedures to achieve soft tissue coverage are mandatory. Another paper addresses the currently accepted indications for the replantation of amputated and partially amputated members, the techniques utilized, and the results that can be achieved.

It is hoped that, given the necessarily limited scope of this booklet, we have provided a useful addition to the trauma literature that will aid the physician in solving the many problems that arise in the treatment of fractures with associated soft tissue injury.

Hannover, February, 1983 H. Tscherne and L. Gotzen

Table of Contents

List of Contributors

Prof. Dr. A. Berger, Klinik für Hand-, Plastische- und Wiederherstellungschirurgie im Krankenhaus Oststadt, Medizinische Hochschule, D-3000 Hannover 51

Dr. V. Echtermeyer, Unfallchirurgische Klinik, Medizinische Hochschule, D-3000 Hannover 61

Priv.-Doz. Dr. N. Haas, Unfallchirurgische Klinik, Medizinische Hochschule, D-3000 Hannover 61

Prof. Dr. G. Muhr, Chirurgische Klinik, Berufsgenossenschaftliche Krankenanstalten „Bergmannsheil", D-4630 Bochum

Priv.-Doz. Dr. H.-J. Oestern, Unfallchirurgische Klinik, Medizinische Hochschule, D-3000 Hannover 61

Dr. D. Rogge, Unfallchirurgische Klinik, Medizinische Hochschule, D-3000 Hannover 61

Dr. M. Rojczyk, Chirurgische Abteilung, Agnes-Karll-Krankenhaus, D-3011 Laatzen

Priv.-Doz. Dr. E.-G. Suren, Unfallchirurgische Klinik, Medizinische Hochschule, D-3000 Hannover 61

Prof. Dr. E. Van der Zypen, Anatomisches Institut der Universität, CH-3012 Bern

Pathophysiology and Classification of Soft Tissue Injuries Associated with Fractures

H.-J. Oestern and H. Tscherne

I. Pathophysiology of Soft Tissue Injuries

The local response to a soft tissue injury has two basic aims:
1. closure of the wound to avoid excessive water and heat loss, and
2. prevention of infection.

1. Local Response to Hemorrhage

All injuries are characterized by some degree of tissue damage and extravasation. Immediately following injury to a blood vessel, platelets bind to collagen and release their phospholipids, which stimulate the *intrinsic coagulation mechanism.* Injured tissue cells release thromboplastin, which activates the *extrinsic coagulation mechanism.*

Platelet adhesion and aggregation lead to the deposition of platelet factor IV and vasoactive amines. Prostaglandin metabolites such as thromboxan A are also secreted, thus augmenting the vasoconstriction produced by the increased amounts of glucocorticoids and catecholamines that are released in response to the trauma.

The vasoconstriction combined with closure of the vessels by the coagulation mechanism creates a hypoxic state in the wound area, leading to acidosis. The proteolytic enzymes released by the aggregating platelets activate the complement system and liberate chemotactic substances which "attract" inflammatory cells, mainly granulocytes (and later mononuclear round cells), to the wound area.

2. Resistance to Infection, Phagocytosis

The function of the macrophages is to inhibit and kill contaminating bacteria, as well as to remove cellular debris from damaged tissue.

Recent investigations suggest that local macrophages play a nutritional role by functioning as the "digestive tract" of the wound. It is also reported (Leibovich, Ross 1975) that macrophages (1) debride injured tissue, (2) process macromolecules to amino acids and sugar, (3) attract other macrophages, (4) signal for further fibroblast replication, (5) stimulate the formation of new blood vessels, and (6) secrete lactate.

Once a neutrophilic granulocyte reaches the damaged tissue, further steps in the phagocytic defense mechanism are initiated. These processes are facilitated by humoral factors called opsonins.

The main components of this system are immunoglobulin G antibodies, which bind to the surface of the bacterium, as well as heat-labile factors which belong to the complement and properdin system and further stimulate this process.

The heat-labile systems fix fragments of complement 3 to the microbial surface via the classic antigen-antibody activated C1, C4, C 2 complement way or via the alternative C3 activation pathway (Gigli, Nelson 1968; Johnston et al. 1969). The opsonins fix the bacterium to the cell wall by combining with receptor molecules on the surface of the phagocyte. Once the phagocyte has fixed the microbe to its surface, it engulfs it with its pseudopodia and digests it.

3. The Importance of Oxygen

Phagocytosis initiates several metabolic processes in the neutrophils that are necessary for their function.

Within seconds after the material is ingested, oxygen consumption within the phagocyte rises to 15–20 times the basal value (Baldridge 1933).

In normal phagocytes, some of the oxygen is enzymatically reduced to superoxide. Superoxide is an unstable molecule that has shown bactericidal activity against clostridia and other organisms which lack the superoxide dismutase that converts superoxide to hydrogen peroxide (Babior 1973). Superoxide is quickly reduced to hydrogen peroxide in the phagosome. Hydrogen peroxide directly kills certain organisms (Karnovsky 1963), and in the presence of myoloperoxidase (MPO and chlorine ions), its antimicrobial activity is greatly increased.

Fibroblast and leukocyte function are depressed by hypoxia (Hunt, Pai 1972; Hunt 1974; Mandell 1974; Hunt et al. 1975). Studies by Hohn et al. (1976) have shown that the number of *Staphylococcus aureus* organisms killed by leukocytes in vitro and in experimental animal wounds increases as the local oxygen tension is raised. From this and other research, it has become clear that soft tissue injuries in hypoxic areas heal poorly. *Ischemic, dessicated tissue cannot be adequately perfused and so is exceedingly susceptible to infection.*

Moreover, granulocytes and macrophages have only a limited capacity for phagocytosis. If they exhaust that capacity by ingesting too much necrotic tissues, their microbicidal capacity is markedly reduced. Hence, *extensive debridement with removal of all necrotic tissue is a highly effective means of preventing infection.*

4. Humoral Mechanisms of Wound Healing

Other substances released in response to tissue injury are mitogenic substances, hydrolases, chemotactic agents, histamine and prostaglandins.

The *mitogenic substances* released by the platelets and damaged tissue promote fibroblast replication and protein biosynthesis.

The *hydrolases* break down cell debris to soluble and diffusible substances. This enzymatic breakdown in turn yields mitogenic and chemotactically active substances which stimulate phagocytosis. However, these materials are rapidly degraded and inactivated by progression of the enzymatic reaction.

Tissue injury also triggers a release of chemotactic substances. One effect of these substances is to attract macrophages and mast cells to the wound margins. Chemotactic substances present in the blood plasma include kallikrein and fibrinopeptide B, which is split off from fibrinogen by the action of thrombin.

Histamine and *prostaglandins* are also released. Both produce an increase in capillary permeability, causing fluid to extravasate into the wound and leading to wound edema.

Edema is necessary for the activation of adventitious cells and for the conversion of fibroblasts to fibrocytes. It can also help lower the concentration of toxic substances in the wound area.

When a soft tissue injury occurs, the processes described above are partly sequential and partly concurrent. Tissue synthesis and lysis complement each other in varying ways. They either cause a progressive degradation of tissue in a setting of hypoxia and acidosis, thus leading to necrosis, or they enable granulation and scar tissue to develop through the formation of proteiglycanes, collagen and elastin.

5. Clinical Relevance

If adequate primary care is to be provided, it is important that the following points be understood:

a) All injuries, whether open or closed, lead to hypoxia in the damaged tissue.
b) Hypoxia and acidosis cause a further increase in vascular permeability.
c) The increased permeability leads to interstitial edema, swelling, and, by raising the interstitial pressure, to an amplification of the hypoxia and acidosis.
d) In severely injured patients with general hypoxia and acidosis, this tissue damage becomes protracted in the periphery.
e) Any mechanical constriction, whether caused by the fascia or skin, causes further deterioration of the metabolic state in the injured tissue, predisposing to infection and hampering wound repair.

Essential to the primary care of any wound, however, is an accurate *evaluation of the soft tissue injury.*

6. Definition of Wound

Lexer (1934) defines a wound as a more or less gaping disruption in the continuity of the outer skin, mucous membranes or organ surfaces. Wounds of the skin can take various forms. An abrasion, for example, is a scraping away of the skin caused by the action of a tangential force. It may be superficial and confined to the epidermis, or it may be deep and involve the corium, depending on the energy of the trauma.

A contusion is a closed injury caused by the transfer of kinetic energy during an impact. It may be confined to the skin or may also involve deeper structures. The rupture of blood vessels within the contused area causes extravasation beneath the skin.

An avulsion or degloving injury occurs when the skin and subcutaneous tissue are stripped away from the underlying muscle and fascia by a tangential force. Large hematomatous areas may result.

A mutilated wound is one in which there is extreme mechanical destruction of tissues, organs or body parts.

Frequently it is not possible to classify a soft tissue injury definitively from an external inspection of the wound. Roentgenograms are helpful in some instances.

7. Roentgenography and Soft Tissue Damage

Extensive displacement, comminution, and roentgenographic changes in soft tissue structures (foreign bodies, air inclusions, soft tissue defects) can in themselves be an indication of the severity of the soft tissue injury.

On the other hand, even a simple-looking fracture may be accompanied by extensive soft tissue damage, because a spontaneous or manual reduction of the fracture at the accident scene can cause initial roentgenographic findings to be deceptive. However, smooth transverse fractures and even segmental fractures of the tibia are usually the result of direct violence and thus will be associated with characteristic soft tissue lesions. In one review of 110 segmental tibial fractures, 50% of the fractures were open, and soft tissue contusions were present in 40% (Mommsen et al., ASIF Collective Study 1980). Segmental fractures have the poorest prognosis of all fractures in terms of union.

8. Soft Tissue Injuries Associated with Closed and Open Fractures

Soft tissue injuries accompanying closed fractures are especially troublesome and often are insufficiently appreciated on account of their occult nature. Even a simple skin contusion over a closed fracture can pose a more complex range of therapeutic and prognostic problems than skin which has been broken by the fractured bone. The main complication of such a contusion is necrosis, which predisposes the tissue to infection. A contaminated, deep abrasion is also highly susceptible to infection due to a breaching of the cutaneous barrier.

In open fractures, the nature and the extent of soft tissue injuries depend upon additional factors as well. Besides the severity of the bony injury, the mechanism of the injury, and the time elapsed between injury and treatment, the level of contamination has a critical bearing on the course and prognosis of the open fracture.

II. Classification of Soft Tissue Injuries

The aim of classifying soft tissue injuries is to describe and grade the injury in the most comprehensive terms possible, so as to guide the surgeon in choosing the appropriate operative tactics.

1. Traditional Classifications of Soft Tissue Injuries

The simple classification of fractures as "open" or "closed" appears to be the only universally accepted scheme. While only a few classifications have been proposed for closed fractures (Tscherne, Brüggemann 1976; Tscherne, Oestern 1982), open fractures have been classified according to a variety of criteria. Allgöwer (1971) recognizes three grades of severity in the open fracture: grade I, in which the skin is pierced from within by a spike of bone; grade II, in which the tissues are contused by violence from without; and grade III, characterized by extensive damage to skin, muscles, blood vessels, nerves and tendons. Gustilo and J.P. Anderson (1976) classify open fractures into three types based upon the extent of the principal injury: type 1 with a skin wound less than 1 cm long; type 2 with a skin lesion more than 1 cm long and with minimal soft tissue damage; and type 3, which may be an open segmental fracture, an open fracture with extensive soft tissue damage, or a traumatic amputation.

The classification of Cauchoix et al. (1965, 1975) is also based essentially on the size of the skin wound. A more differentiated approach is taken by L.D. Anderson (1971), who classifies open fractures according to the extent of avascular and necrotic changes and the amount of foreign material in the wound. Type 1 is a punctate wound with little soft tissue damage, type 2 is a large wound with a small amount of avascular or devitalized soft tissue, and type 3 is an extensive wound with massive soft tissue necrosis and contamination by foreign material.

On the whole, the schemes proposed today seem unable to provide a definitive classification of the soft tissue injuries that accompany fractures. This inadequacy prompted us to devise our own system for the classification of open and closed fractures.

2. Own Classification

In our system, closed and open fractures are each classified into four grades of severity (Table 1) as follows:

Table 1. Classification of soft tissue injuries in closed and open fractures according to soft tissue damage, fracture severity and contamination

Classification	Skin open + closed –	Soft tissue damage	Fracture severity mild + mod. ++ sev. +++	Contamination
Fr. C 0	–	–	+	–
C I	–	+	+ to ++	–
C II	–	++	+ to +++	–
C III	–	+++	+ to +++	–
Fr. O I	+	+	+ to ++	+
O II	+	++	+ to +++	++
O III	+	+++	+ to +++	+++
O IV	+	+++	+ to +++	+ to +++

a) Closed Fractures

Grade 0 closed fractures (Fr. C 0): Soft tissue damage is absent or negligible. The fracture is caused by indirect violence and has a simple configuration (Fig. 1). Torsion fractures of the tibia in skiers are typical of this category.

Grade I closed fractures (Fr. C I): There is a superficial abrasion or contusion caused by fragment pressure from within. The fracture itself is of a mild to moderately severe configuration (Fig. 2). A typical example is the pronation fracture-dislocation of the ankle joint, in which soft tissue lesions are caused by pressure from the fractured margin of the medial malleolus.

Grade II closed fracture (Fr. C II): There is a deep, contaminated abrasion associated with localized skin or muscle contusion from direct trauma (Fig. 3). Impending compartment syndrome is included in this category. Generally there has been direct violence producing a moderately severe to severe fracture configuration. Segmental "bumper" fractures of the tibia are an example. Given the mechanism of injury, the soft tissue lesions must be at least Fr. C I but are usually Fr. C II.

Grade III closed fracture (Fr. C III): The skin is extensively contused or crushed, and muscle damage may be severe. Other criteria for this category are subcutaneous avulsions, decompensated compartment syndrome, and rupture of a major blood vessel associated with a closed fracture (Fig. 4). The fracture configuration is severe or comminuted. The contu-

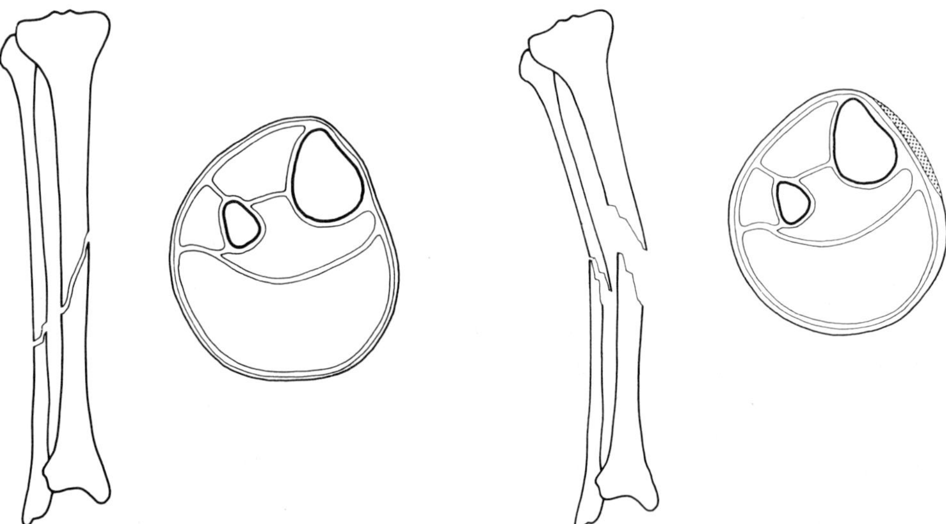

Fig. 1 (left). Grade 0 closed fracture (Fr. C 0): Simple fracture configuration with little or no soft tissue injury

Fig. 2 (right). Grade I closed fracture (Fr. C I): Superficial abrasion (*shaded area*), mild to moderately severe fracture configuration

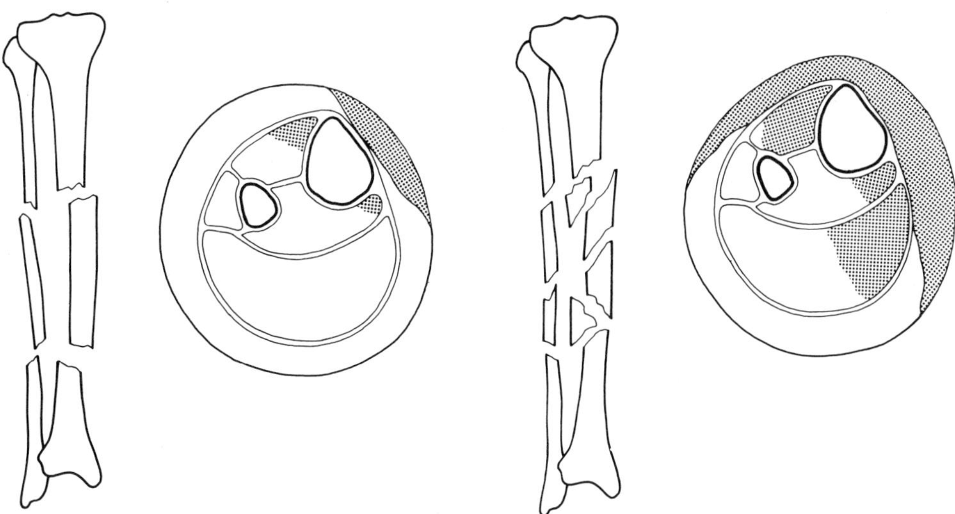

Fig. 3 (left). Grade II closed fracture (Fr. C II): Deep, contaminated abrasion with local contusional damage to skin or muscle (*shaded area*), moderately severe fracture configuration (e.g., closed segmental fracture of the tibial shaft)

Fig. 4 (right). Grade III closed fracture (Fr. C III): Extensive contusion or crushing of skin or destruction of muscle (*shaded area*), severe fracture

sional damage makes treatment of the soft tissue injuries more difficult than in grade III open fractures.

b) Open Fractures

The evaluation and treatment of open fractures is governed both by the extent of soft tissue injuries and by the level of wound contamination. The primary concern is *not* the size of the skin wound, but the degree of soft tissue damage and extent of muscle contusions. Consequently, it may not be possible to make a definitive classification until the wound has been explored.

Grade I open fracture (Fr. O I): Open wound with little or no skin contusion. Bacterial contamination is negligible. Usually the skin is pierced by only one bone fragment of variable length. Generally the fracture is of a mild configuration.

Grade II open fracture (Fr. O II): Open wound with circumscribed skin and soft tissue contusions and moderate contamination. The severity of the fracture is variable.

Grade III open fracture (Fr. O III): Open, heavily contaminated wound with extensive soft tissue destruction, often with associated vascular and nerve lesions. Any open fracture with ischemia and extensive comminution. Gunshot wounds and open, contaminated fractures due to farm injuries are included in this category. Due to the high risk of infection, all fractures involving injury to the major extremital arteries should be classified as Fr. O III.

Grade IV open fracture (Fr. O IV): Total or subtotal amputation. According to the Replantation Committee of the International Society for Reconstructive Microsurgery (Biemer 1981), a subtotal amputation is characterized by division of the major anatomic structures, particularly the major vascular connections, with complete ischemia. The soft tissue envelope may be intact for no more than one-fourth of its circumference. If major anatomic connections are still present and there is clear evidence of a residual blood flow (revascularization), the injury is classified as a grade III open fracture.

Though a more detailed classification of grade IV open fractures is useful for purposes of replantation (micro- and macroreplantation, condition of amputated part, duration of ischemia, coexisting injuries, etc.), we have refrained from this in order to keep our classification as simple as possible. For similar reasons, total and subtotal amputations were not placed into separate categories.

References

1. Allgöwer M (1971) Weichteilprobleme und Infektrisiko der Osteosynthese. Langenbecks Arch Chir 329:1127
2. Anderson LD (1971) Fractures. In: Campbells Operative Orthopaedics. Mosby, St. Louis
3. Babior BM, Kipnes RS, Curnutte JT (1973) Biological defense mechanisms. The production by leukocytes of superoxide, a potential bactericidal agent. J Clin Invest 52: 741
4. Baldridge CW, Gerard RW (1933) The extra respiration of pathocytosis. Am J Physiol 103:235
5. Biemer E, Duspiva W (1980) Rekonstruktive Gefäßchirurgie. Springer, Berlin Heidelberg New York
6. Cauchoix J, Lagneau P, Boulez P (1965) Traitement des fractures ouvertes de jambe. Resultats de 234 cas observes entre le 1er janvier 1955 et le 12 juin 1964. Ann Chir 19:1520
7. Cauchoix J, Duparc J, Boulez P (1975) Traitement des fractures ouvertes des jambe. Med Acta Chir 83:811
8. Gigli I, Nelson RA Jr (1968) Complement dependent immune phagocytosis. Exp Cell Res 51:45
9. Gustilo B, Anderson JP (1976) Prevention of infection in the treatment of one thousand and twenty-five open fractures of long bones. J Bone Joint Surg 58A:453
10. Hohn DC, MacKay RD, Halliday B, Hunt ThK (1976) Effect of O_2 tension and microbucudak function of leukocytes in wounds and in vitro. Surg Forum 27:18
11. Hohn DC (1977) Leukocyte phagocytic function and dysfunction. Surg Gynecol Obstet 144:99
12. Hunt TK, Pai MP (1972) The effect of varying ambient oxygen tensions on wound metabolism and collagen synthesis. Surg Gynecol Obstet 135:561
13. Hunt TK, Linsey M, Grislis G, Sonne M, Jawetz E (1975) The effect of different ambient oxygen tensions on wound infection. Ann Surg 181:35
14. Johnston RB Jr, Klemper MR, Alper CA et al. (1969) The enhancement of bacterial phagocytosis by serum; the role of complement components and two co-factors. J Exp Med 129:1275
15. Karnovsky ML (1962) Metabolic basis of phagicytic activity. Physiol Rev 42:143
16. Knapp U (1981) Die Wunde. Thieme, Stuttgart
17. Leibovich SJ, Ross R (1975) The role of the macrophage in wound repair. Am J Pathol 78:71

18. Mandell GL (1974) Bactericidal activity of aerobic and anaerobic polymorphonuclear-neutrophils. Infect Immun 9:337
19. Mommsen U, Stammer HJ, Jungbluth KH (1980) Der Unterschenkeletagenbruch. Unfallchir 6:178
20. Rutherford RB, Ross R (1976) Platelet factors stimulate fibroblasts and smooth muscle cells quiescent in serum to proliferate. J Cell Biol 69:196
21. Schweiberer L, van de Berg A, Dambe LT (1970) Das Verhalten der intraossären Gefäße nach Osteosynthese der frakturierten Tibia des Hundes. Therapiewoche 20:1330
22. Tscherne H, Brüggemann H (1976) Die Weichteilbehandlung bei Osteosynthesen, insbesondere bei offenen Frakturen. Unfallheilkunde 79:467
23. Tscherne H, Oestern HJ (1982) Die Klassifizierung des Weichteilschadens bei offenen und geschlossenen Frakturen. Unfallheilkunde 85:111

The Management of Open Fractures

H. Tscherne

Introduction

Open fractures are a serious surgical emergency. They demand urgent yet thoughful intervention on the part of the surgeon. The tactics employed during the first hours can make the difference between complete recovery and a life of disability. Soft tissue problems are the decisive factor with regard to treatment. They may be either traumatic or posttraumatic in origin; that is, they may be caused by the violence of the injury or may result from errors and problems of indication, primary care or postoperative management.

Over the past 50 years there have been four major eras in the treatment of open fractures: the era of life preservation, the era of limb preservation, the era of infection avoidance, and the era of function preservation. The first of these, which might also be called the preantiseptic era, lasted well into the 20th Century. During this period, loss of life was a very real danger for patients with open fractures. At the German Surgeon's Congress of 1878, Richard von Volkmann reported a mortality rate of 38.5% for this type of injury. Theodor Billroth (1866) remarked: "I can state from my own experience that the most remarkable operative cure has never given me such satisfaction as the successful treatment of a severe open fracture."

This comment is understandable, for in Billroth's series of 93 patients with open fractures of the tibia, there were 36 deaths and 28 amputations. The second era, that of limb preservation, roughly encompassed the war years and was characterized by a very high incidence of surgical amputations.

The third era, lasting until the mid-1960s, saw much progress made toward avoiding the most frequent and feared complication of open wounds, infection. Secondary infection by hospital organisms was a more serious problem than primary wound contamination at the time of the injury. Even today, the avoidance of infection upon admission to the hospital and of infection secondary to soft tissue necrosis is a major concern in the management of open fractures.

Around 1965, progress in fracture treatment ushered in the fourth era, that of function preservation. Nowadays, highest priority is given to maintaining the functional integrity of an injured extremity, even at the cost of infection. The citizen of today makes ever-increasing demands of our society. Even with a severe open fracture, he not only expects that the bone will heal, but insists upon a complete return of normal function to the extremity.

Although the specific management of open fractures has varied over the years, a definite trend has emerged in favor of aggressive wound debridement with excision of all dead and devascularized tissues, definitive fracture treatment employing internal or external fixation, and delayed wound closure (Tscherne et al. 1967; Tscherne 1969; Allgöwer 1971; Burri 1974; Tscherne, Brüggemann 1974, 1976; Tscherne 1975, 1977, 1981).

Principles of Treatment

A well-defined therapeutic concept is essential to the successful treatment of open fractures. The steps outlined below, arranged in temporal sequence, provide a useful guide to management (Table 1).

Table 1. Management of open fractures

	Care setting
1. First aid	Accident scene ↓
2. Primary in-hospital care	Emergency room ↓
3. Preparations for surgery	OR or preparation room ↓
4. Surgical treatment	OR ↓
5. Postoperative care	ICU

1. Prehospital Care

The cardinal rule at the accident scene is to avoid further soft tissue injury (Fig. 1). We strongly recommend that the fractures should be reduced on the scene, as this will relieve pressure on the injured, ischemic soft tissues. Swelling and the spread of hematoma are controlled by placing a sterile dressing over the wound and immobilizing the extremity in a pneumatic splint (Fig. 2).

External bleeding is best controlled with a sterile compressive dressing. In rare instances it may be necessary to apply a sterile hemostat to control arterial hemorrhage. A tourniquet is indicated only in the face of unmanageable hemorrhage or traumatic amputation, for even a properly applied occlusion dressing or penumatic tourniquet will produce ischemia of the peripheral vessels, which in turn promotes infection.

As emergency rescue services are expanded and improved, an increasing number of open fractures are being treated on the scene by trained emergency physicians. In our practice, for example, 59% of the open fractures seen by us have already received field treatment within about 20 minutes postinjury from one of our residents who accompanied the rescue vehicle to the scene. The benefits of this early care are substantial (Rojczyk, Tscherne 1982), as Table 2 indicates: a 3.5% infection rate when primary care was administered by air ambulance personnel, as opposed to a 22.2% infection rate in patients who reached the trauma center by way of another hospital within 10 hours postinjury. In the latter case, every fifth patient with an open fracture developed an infection. Naturally, the time factor has a significant bearing on the end result regardless of the quality of primary care.

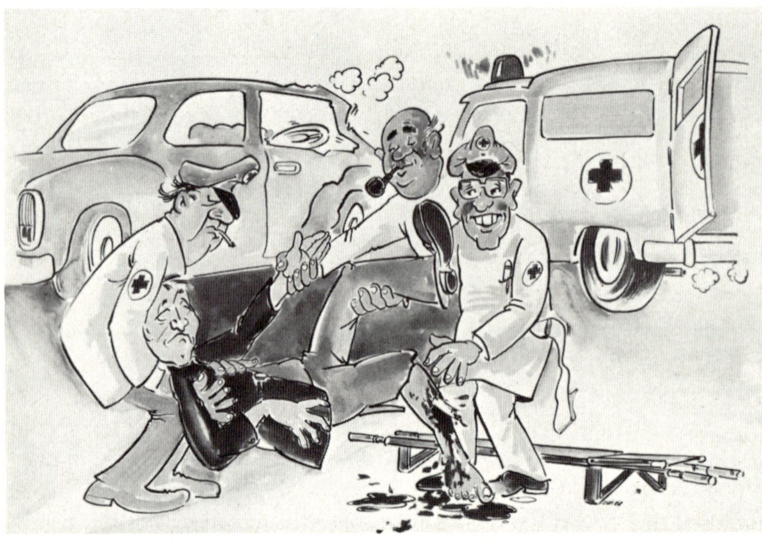

Fig. 1. Careless handling of the patient at the accident scene potentiates soft tissue injuries

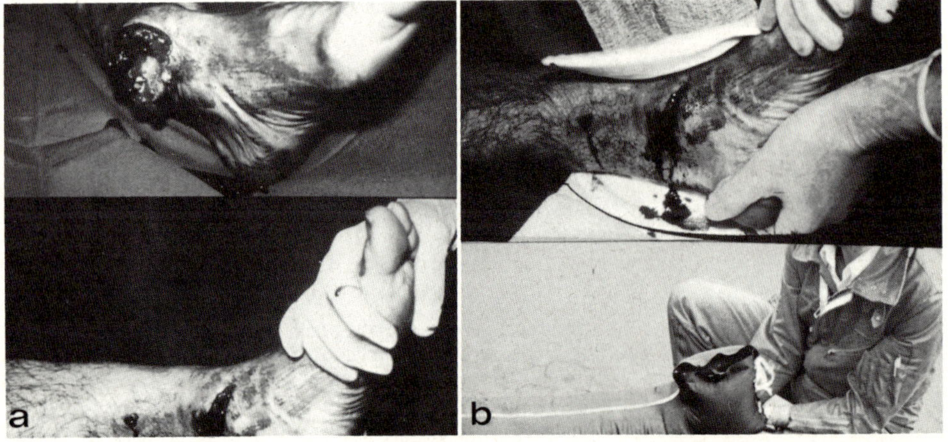

Fig. 2a, b. Markedly displaced fractures should be reduced on the scene. An open fracture-dislocation of the ankle joint is realigned by traction and countertraction (**a**). The wound is covered with a sterile dressing, and the limb is immobilized in a pneumatic splint (**b**)

2. Initial In-Hospital Care

Upon admission, the sterile field dressing should not be removed for inspection of the wound. Both the dressing and splint are left in place throughout the period of preoperative care. Because the majority of open fractures are the result of extreme violence, many

Table 2. Infection rates for various modes of primary care

Primary care		Infection rate	
Rescue helicopter	(n = 86)	3	(3.5%)
Ambulance with physician aboard	(n = 22)	2	(9.1%)
Ground rescue vehicle	(n = 41)	5	(12.2%)
Inter hospital transfer within 10 hrs postinjury	(n = 45)	10	(22.2%)

patients will present with multiple injuries. Treatment for asphyxia, blood loss, shock and other life-threatening conditions must take precedence over all else. Once life-threatening problems have been corrected and the patient is in stable condition a more definitive diagnostic evaluation may be made, with emphasis placed upon speed, accuracy and thoroughness. Even at this stage, however, the emergency dressing should not be disturbed. Nor should the wound be inspected or palpated by the entire emergency room staff to determine whether and in what manner the fracture communicates with the outside environment (Fig. 3).

On the other hand, it is imperative that the limb be closely examined for evidence of adequate blood supply. If no peripheral pulses are detected, it is important to examine for capillary flow. Often a good peripheral capillary flow can supply enough blood to ensure survival of the limb despite absence of the peripheral pulses. The simplest test is to depress the nail bed of the finger or toe and watch for capillary refill following release. Skin color

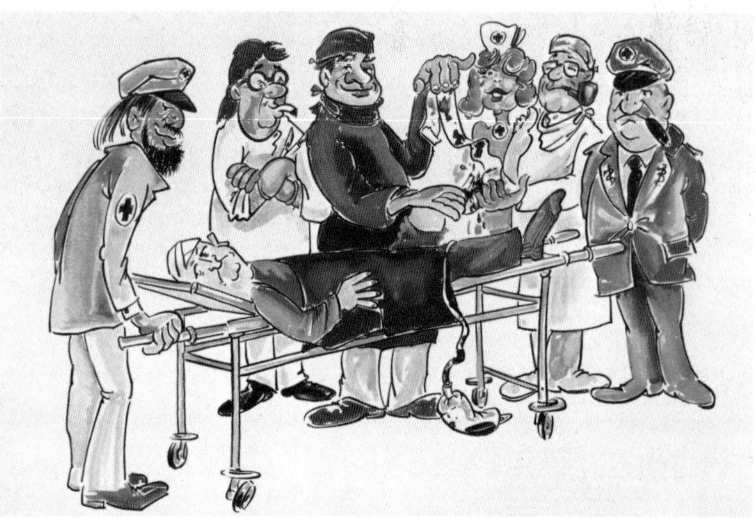

Fig. 3. Needless risks are created when all personnel in ER are allowed to view or examine the wound. The sterile dressing applied in the field should not be removed

and temperature are additional guides. The peripheral vascular flow may also be evaluated by means of ultrasonography or, if necessary, by angiography.

The joints adjacent to the open fracture are carefully examined so that coexisting injuries will not be overlooked. These joints are included in the roentgenographic study. Insufficient roentgenograms should not be accepted. It is essential that all bony injuries be well documented before the operation begins. Occasionally it is useful to obtain oblique roentgenograms of the fracture site so that the extent of the osseous injury can be better appreciated.

Often it is impossible to obtain a complete history. Nevertheless, every effort should be made to establish at least the time, cause and mechanism of the accident. The clothing over the injury should be inspected to rule out the presence of cloth fragments in the wound.

Preparations for Surgery

From the emergency room, the patient is taken to the operating room or preparation room, where, under aseptic conditions, the primary dressing may at last be removed. The importance of leaving the sterile field dressing in place is illustrated in Table 3. The surgeon is now able to make a definitive evaluation of the soft tissue injury. On the basis of this examination and roentgenographic findings, the tactics of the operation are planned. If a grade III open fracture is present, the surgeon will have to determine whether or not primary amputation is indicated. With a grade IV open fracture, it mus be decided whether replantation is feasible.

In cases of severe crush injury or neurovascular trauma, the costs of reconstructive surgery to salvage the extremity should always be weighed against the degree of function that may be anticipated. In critically- or multiple-injured patients, the decision to amputate is simplified. Under no circumstances should the life of these patients be endangered by prolonged major surgery.

Surgical preparation of the injured area begins by shaving the surrounding skin with a sterile disposable razor and cleansing it with a brush and povidone-iodine solution. Dirty bone fragments visible in the wound are also scrubbed. Then the wound is flushed repeatedly with Ringer's solution. This irrigation washes bacteria from the wound while also removing small blood clots and necrotic debris from the muscle, bone and fat. The entire limb is again disinfected before a sterile drape is applied (Fig. 4).

For fractures with soft tissue injury, a tourniquet should not be used. However, it is wise to have a tourniquet on hand in case it is needed to control intraoperative bleeding.

Table 3. Infection rates of open fractures, with and without continuous sterile coverage from accident scene to operating room

With sterile dressing n = 116	Without sterile dressing n = 77
Infection rate	
5 (4.3%)	15 (19.2%)

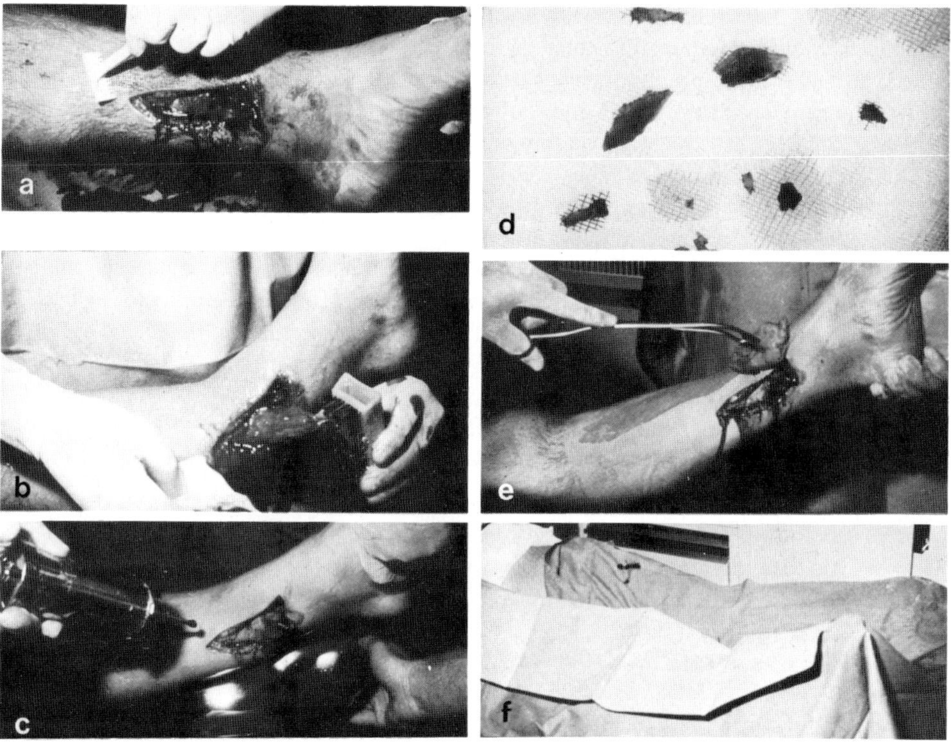

Fig. 4a–f. Preparations for surgery: The area is shaved with a sterile disposable razor (**a**) and cleansed with a brush (**b**). The wound is irrigated (**c**) to flush out bone fragments and foreign material (**d**). The skin is then painted with antiseptic solution (**e**). The extremity is wrapped in a sterilized cloth before entering the OR (**f**)

4. Operative Treatment

Debridement

The operative technique is dictated by the severity of the soft tissue injury. Wound debridement is unnecessary for grade I open fractures in which there is simply an inside-to-outside puncture wound caused by indirect violence. However, it is still necessary to account for all clothing over the fracture site so that foreign material in the wound may be ruled out. A small perforating wound is sparingly debrided and left open. The fracture is treated conservatively as a closed injury, or operative fixation is carried out.

For all other grades of open fracture, a meticulous debridement is indicated. Living tissue offers the best defense against infection.

The majority of infections are distinct pathophysiologically from other bacterial infections such as phlegmon, erysipelas and abscess. A hyperacute inflammation that spreads rapidly to surrounding tissues causing purulent liquefaction is not characteristic of the infected open fracture. Infections following open fractures tend to be less a result of primary bacterial contamination than of local tissue hypoxia or anoxia. Next to hematomas, tissues that are poorly perfused or devitalized offer the best medium for bacterial growth (remember: debridement does not completely eliminate microorganisms but only decreases their count). Necrosis will allow bacterial proliferation to proceed at a more or less rapid pace. The infection takes a protracted course and often is unaccompanied by obvious general signs of inflammation. It is common for primarily clean wounds to become infected secondarily, even by the hematogenous route. We have seeen several instances of blood-borne infection of fracture hematomas in intensive-care patients with closed injuries. The most frequent causes of infection in patients with open fractures are the following:

- incomplete excision of poorly vascularized tissue, especially muscle, skin and bone;
- inadequate hemostasis and hematoma evacuation, and insuffient drainage of wound discharges and wound hematoma;
- devascularization of primarily viable tissue;
- large metallic fixation devices implanted under poorly vascularized tissue;

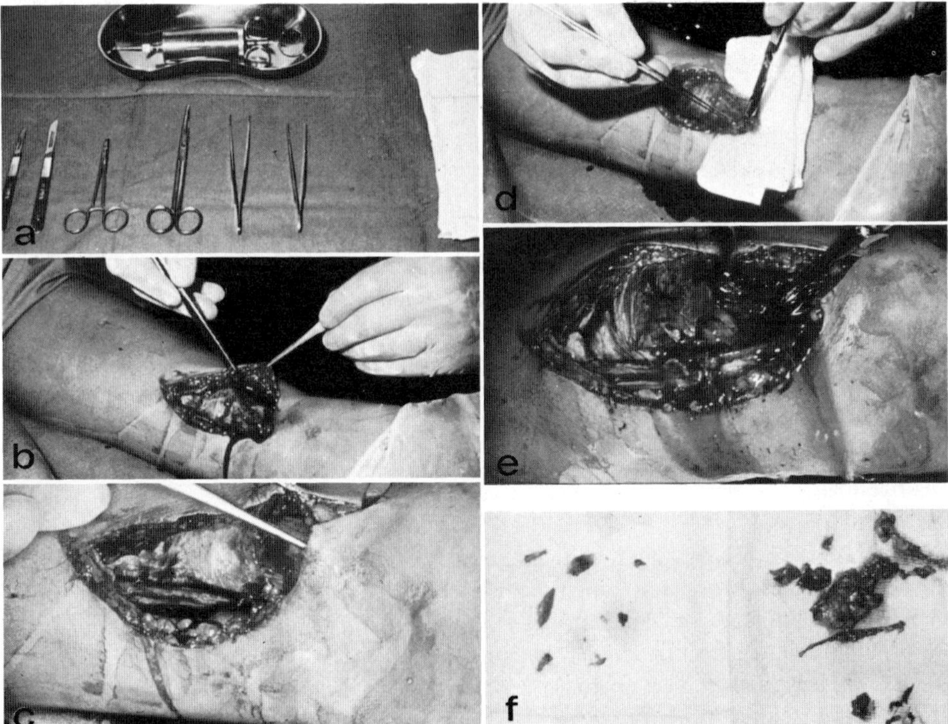

Fig. 5a–f. Wound debridement. Relatively few instruments are needed (**a**). The wound margins are sparingly excised (**b**). Often the primary wound will have to be extended (**c**). The bone and periosteum are included in debridement (**d**). Occasionally the bone must be "freshened" with a ronguer or chisel (**e**). Flushed-out cortical bone fragments are shown at the left, and excised soft tissues at the right (**f**)

- wound closure under tension;
- failure to recognize compartment syndrome.

By now, the fundamental importance of radically excising all devitalized tissue should be appreciated (Fig. 5). In most cases the exposure needed for this debridement can be gained only by extending the primary wound. Thus, the surgical approach and the optimum placement of internal fixation material under cover of viable tissue must be established before the operation commences. The surgical approach is of crucial importance. When extending the wound, the surgeon should try to reconcile the preexisting wound with one of the standard orthopedic approaches. The latter run in a longitudinal direction, and all secondary incisions should be longitudinally oriented.

Transverse, oblique and longitudinal wounds should be incorporated into the standard incisions if their localizations permit (e.g., wounds over the anterior tibial margin, lateral wounds of the thigh). If the primary wounds cannot be incorporated into any of the standard incisions, then internal fixation, if indicated, will have to be done through a separate standard incision. Large wounds, especially of the upper arm and thigh, that are situated away from standard lines of incision may in themselves afford sufficient access for stabilizing the fracture.

A separate incision is recommended if the bridge of skin between the primary wound and proposed incision is 5 cm or more in width. With extensive wounds, care must be taken not to exceed a ratio of 3 : 1 between the length and width of the skin bridge. It is best to avoid creating skin flaps if at all possible.

Internal fixation material may also be introduced through one or two separate longitudinal incisions placed at least 5 cm from the primary wound. If the traumatic wound is oriented at right angles to the limb axis, a V-shaped extensile incision may be utilized, taking care that the wound angles are no smaller than 110°.

The skin margins of the wound are excised sparingly or not at all. With a degloving injury, it is best to remove the subcutaneous fat from the avulsed tissue and convert the skin to a full-thickness pedicle graft.

During debridement, all cavities within the wound must be exposed and freed of foreign material. Bleeding is meticulously controlled. The viability of all tissues should be assessed as they are exposed. In the case of muscle, the "4 C's" provide a useful criterial for viability (Fig. 6):

- consistency
- conctractility
- color
- capacity to bleed.

A muscle that bleeds when cut and contracts when touched is almost certainly viable (Heppenstall 1980). It is best to resect muscle whose viability is doubtful. The alternative is to leave questionable muscle in place and return the patient to the operating room two to three days later for a second look.

Exposure of the fracture should be developed as atraumatically as possible so that the blood supply to the fragments is not compromised. Hohmann retractors and other hook-like instruments that encircle the bone should not be used on account of their denuding effect. Grossly dirty bone is freshened, and indriven foreign bodies are removed with a chisel or ronguer (Fig. 7). Loose pieces of cortical bone count as potential sequestra and

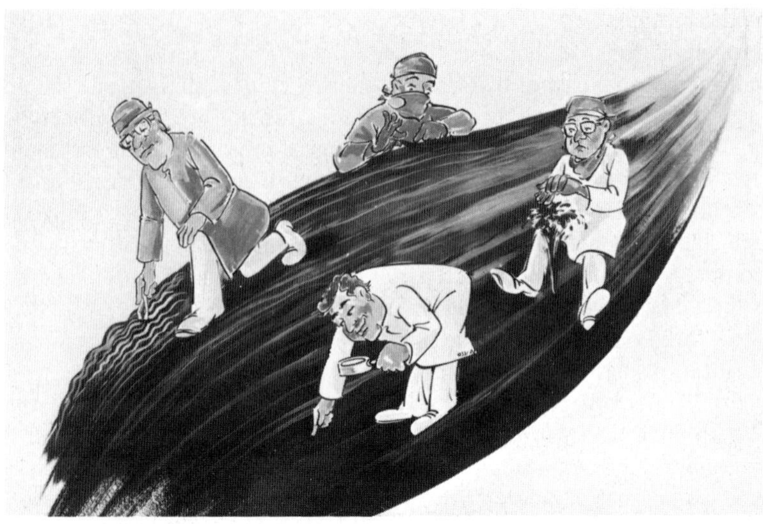

Fig. 6. Determining muscle viability. A viable muscle contracts when touched, has a soft, "fleshy" consistency, is reddish-brown in color, and bleeds actively

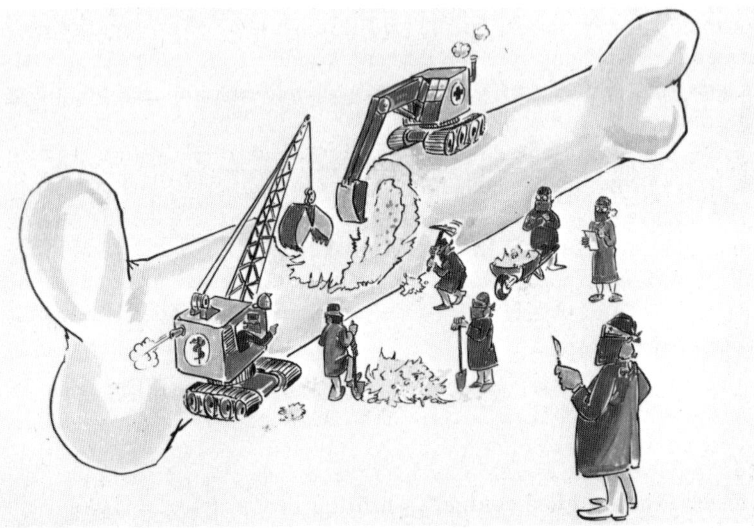

Fig. 7. Radical debridement of the bone is an essential part of the wound debridement routine

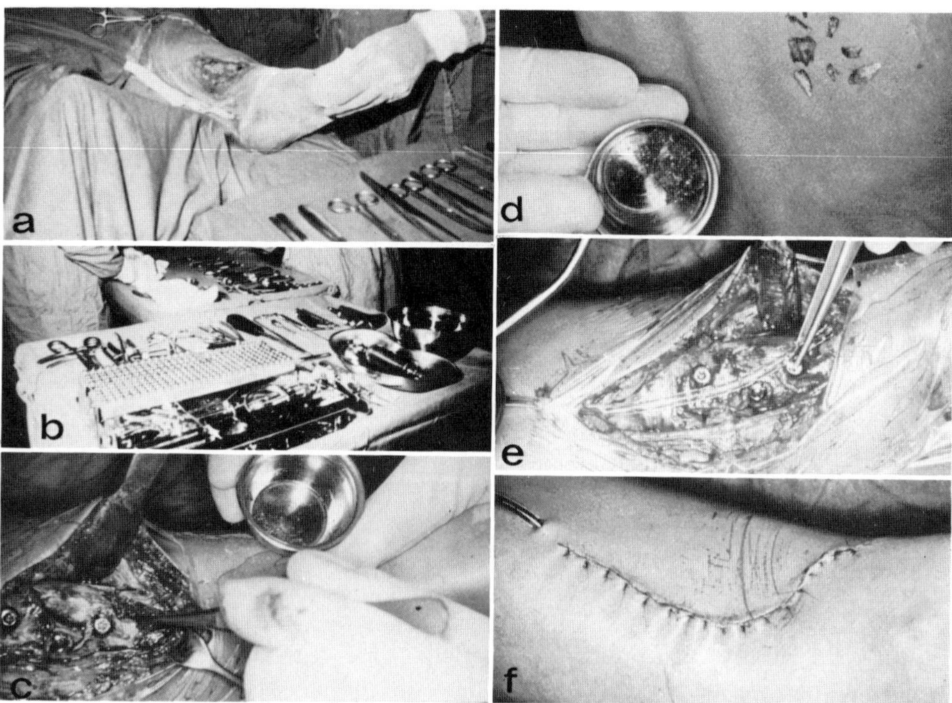

Fig. 8. For the second stage of the operation, the entire wound area is redraped, surgical attire is changed, and new instruments are introduced (**a**, **b**). The fracture should be stabilized with a minimum of implant material (**c**). Isolated cortical fragments are removed and replaced with autologous cancellous bone (**d**). Suction drains are inserted into all wound cavities (**e**). Primary closure without soft tissue tension (**f**). The knots of the Donati-Allgöwer sutures are tied over the wound edge that has the better vascularity

should be extracted unless, for mechanical reasons, it is deemed necessary to incorporate them into the fixation to enhance stability.

During the operation the wound is irrigated repeatedly with Betadine or Ringer's solution. Following the debridement, all surgical instruments and attire are changed, and the wound is redraped as for a new operation (Fig. 8).

The benefits of this routine are demonstrated in a continuous series of 199 open fractures (Rojczyk 1981) (Table 4). As the Table shows, the number of positive smears decreases markedly from initial contamination by the trauma to the end of the operation. (Note, however, that only 22 of the 199 open fractures were primarily contaminated with virulent organisms.)

Table 4. Bacterial contamination of 199 open fractures. The 1st smear was taken at the scene or upon admission, the 2nd following wound debridement, and the 3rd just prior to wound closure

	1st smear	2nd smear	3rd smear
Saprophytes	119	51	14
Staph. epid.	43	15	7
Staph. aur.	10	4	3
Pseud. aerug.	3	3	2
E. coli	8	6	4
Enterobacter	1	1	0
Proteus	0	0	1
Sterile	49	129	168

Stabilization of the Fracture

Once the wound has been satisfactorily debrided, attention is turned toward treating the fracture itself. The benefits of complete immobilization in fracture therapy can no longer be a matter of doubt. Because the majority of these fractures are inherently unstable, even a good primary reduction cannot preclude subsequent slipping of the fragments, leading to pressure on damaged tissues, necrosis, and secondary infection. Optimum conditions of soft tissue healing are ensured only by stable fixation of the fractured bone. The central importance of this principle has been fully appreciated only in the most recent era of open fracture treatment. What once was looked upon as a fundamental error is today considered a *sine qua non* in the successful management of open fractures. Far from increasing the risk of infection, the complete mechanical neutralization of the fracture prevents the development of soft tissue necrosis and encourages wound healing.

We feel that operative fracture stabilization may be dispensed with only in cases where, owing to a minimum of muscular and periosteal damage, the fracture is reasonably stable and can be adequately immobilized by conservative means (e.g., humeral and tibial shaft fractures, periarticular fractures).

In selecting the appropriate method of operative fixation, numerous factors must be considered (see Gotzen, Haas; Rogge). In all cases the surgeon should implant only the minimum amount of fixation material that is consistent with the goal of rigid fixation.

Great care must be taken that metal implants are placed under cover of viable tissue. Implants, tendons, nerves and blood vessels should always be covered by well-perfused soft parts. In the case of the tibia, the lateral aspect of the bone is generally the best site for applying plate fixation. Medial plating is rarely advised, and many bone infections can be traced directly to medial plating with subsequent soft tissue necrosis (Fig. 9).

For open shaft fractures of the upper extremity and femur, we prefer stable internal fixation by compression plating. Only in extreme situations, such as gunshot injuries, do we favor external fixation over plating. For biomechanical reasons we do not advocate intramedullary nailing of the upper extremity under any circumstances (Tscherne 1972, 1976; Tscherne, Oestern 1974). In the lower extremity, the criteria for intramedullary nailing with little or no reaming of the medullary canal are explained by Gotzen and Haas

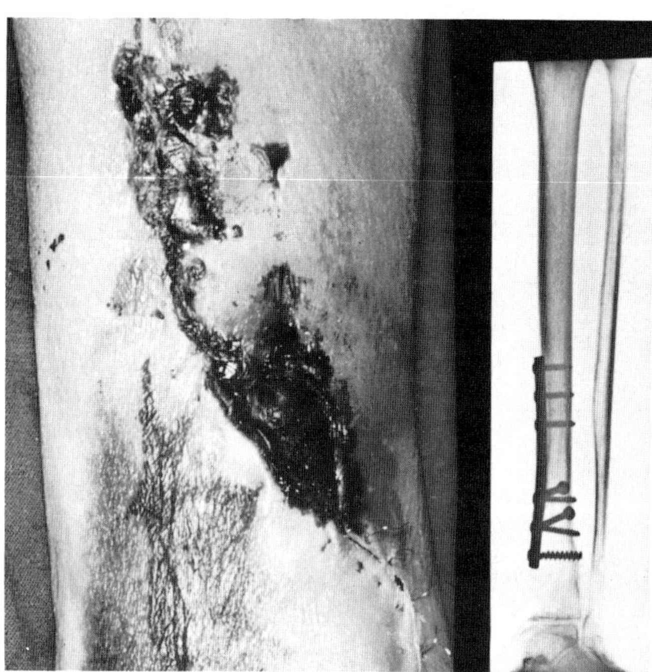

Fig. 9. Open tibial fracture with severe crushing of soft tissues on the medial side. The plate position is incorrect as shown, for it violates the rule that implants must be covered by healthy soft tissue

(p. 53), who also address the problems associated with the operative treatment of tibial fractures in general.

When osseous defects are present, primary or secondary bone grafting is required (Fig. 10). Grafts of autologous cancellous bone heal better than loose, devascularized cortical fragments that are left in place at operation. In the presence of extensive defects and in polytraumatized patients, the prospects of graft healing are improved if the grafting is deferred for 2–3 weeks. After operative fixation is completed, the adjacent joints should be tested for ligamentous stability, since capsular and other ligamentous injuries frequently escape preoperative diagnosis. This is especially common with knee and ankle joint injuries associated with fractures of the femur and tibia.

Vascular Injuries

When vascular damage is present, operative fixation of the accompanying fracture (especially diaphyseal fractures) is a necessity. This raises the question of priorities. It is vital that ischemic time be kept to an absolute minimum. If the circulation cannot be reestablished quickly by means of an intraluminal shunt, then vascular repairs must take precedence over all other measures. Many surgeons in Central Europe stabilize the fracture first before

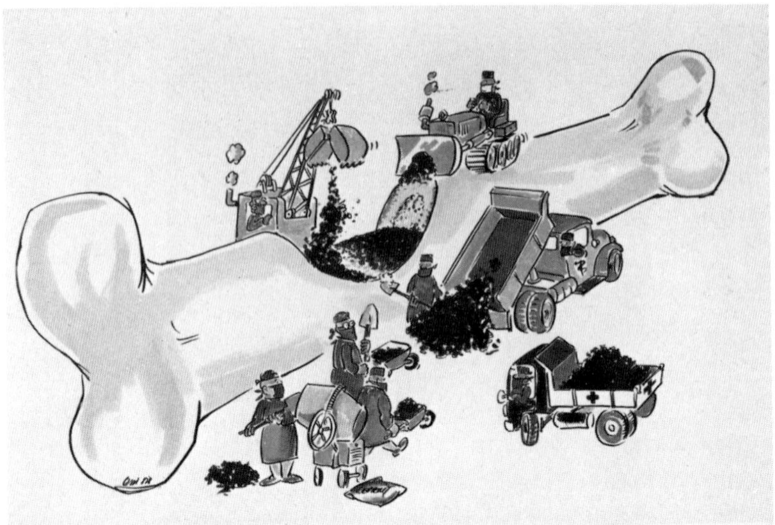

Fig. 10. Osseous defects are packed with autologous cancellous bone. Homologous bone is not utilized in open fractures. Cancellous grafts are also used to bridge zones of devitalized bone

undertaking vascular repairs. We feel that this approach is justified only in exceptional cases. Even the most rapid operative fixation consumes valuable minutes, prolongs ischemic time, and exacerbates the risk of functional loss. After vascular repairs have been completed, the orthopedic surgeon must be able to work on the bone with a minimum of traumatization so that the vascular sutures are not destroyed.

Wound Closure

Subsequent wound treatment following debridement and fixation is of critical importance. It must be understood that the pressure within the tissues rises significantly during the

Table 5. Wound closure

Initial care
Primary closure
Open wound treatment
Synthetic skin
Secondary care
Secondary suture
Split-thickness skin graft
Distant pedicle flaps
Local muscle of myocutaneous flaps
Free tissue transfer with microvascular anatomosis

immediate postoperative period as a result of wound edema. To prevent compartment syndrome, it is important that torn or incised fasciae be left unsutured. Longitudinal and transverse fasciotomies should be made over endangered muscle compartments. Suction drains are inserted in sufficient numbers to reach all recesses of the wound.

Any wound that cannot be closed without tension using atraumatic sutures should be left open. Closure in this situation would inevitably lead to skin and soft tissue necrosis as a result of posttraumatic edema and circulatory impairment (Fig. 11).

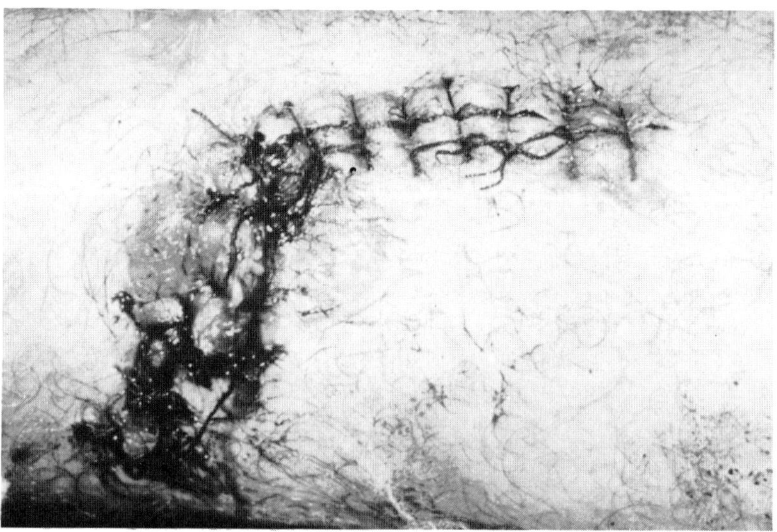

Fig. 11. Skin sutures tied under tension choke the blood supply to the wound edges and adjacent skin, predisposing to necrosis and secondary infection

Primary Wound Closure

Conditions must be ideal for this type of management to be carried out. It may be performed only if the following criteria are met (Heppenstall 1980):

- The blood supply to the affected extremity is essentially normal.
- All dead tissue has been eliminated, and the degree of primary wound contamination is minimal.
- The surgeon is able to close the wound without tension and without significant dead space.

  The dreaded "3 D's":

  dead bone
  dead tissue
  dead space

  are the greatest enemies of an open fracture.

- Primary wound closure may be unsuitable for multiple injury patients with poor compensation of vital organ systems. The decreased oxygen delivery to the wound will delay healing and increase proneness to infection under conditions of relative hypoxia.

In some cases relaxing incisions are very helpful in obtaining coverage of soft tissue defects. With a longitudinal defect over the anterior tibia, for example, a posterior relaxing incision will enable a tension-free closure to be achieved. The relaxing incision of Picot (Fig. 12) is effective only if it encompasses the entire lower leg. After the fascia is incised, medial and lateral soft tissue flaps are developed and advanced toward the front of the limb. Even extensive anterior defects can be closed in this fashion. The skin defect left by the incision remains open and is closed directly by secondary suture or in stages with Steri strips.

Synthetic skin: For the past six years we have used synthetic skin routinely for the primary coverage of skin defects. Epigard, a product of Parke Davis, is a synthetic wound dressing which consists of a layer of polyurethane foam backed by a Teflon film. The microporous Teflon film allows adequate ventilation of the wound but is impervious to bacteria, plasma and exudate. Wound discharges collect in the cavities of the polyurethane foam and coagulate there.

Because Epigard is a dressing, it must be changed at regular intervals (daily or every other day). At this time the wound may be inspected for evidence of necrosis or hematoma. Often, further approximation of the wound margins can also be obtained when the new dressing is applied. After edema has subsided, the wound is closed by secondary suture or covered with simple skin grafts (Rojczyk 1981; Weller et al. 1981) (Figs. 13 and 14).

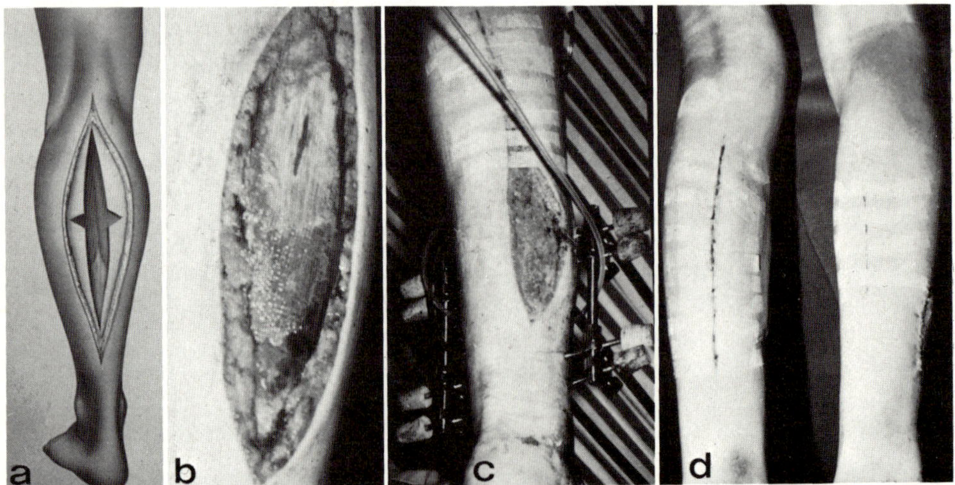

Fig. 12a–d. Picot's relaxing incision for closing longitudinal defects over the anterior tibia. A cruciate fasciotomy is performed, and the medial and lateral soft tissue flaps are mobilized to cover the area of skin loss (**a**). The relaxing incision is left open (**b**). Several days later the defect may be narrowed with Steri strips (**c**) or closed by secondary suture (**d**)

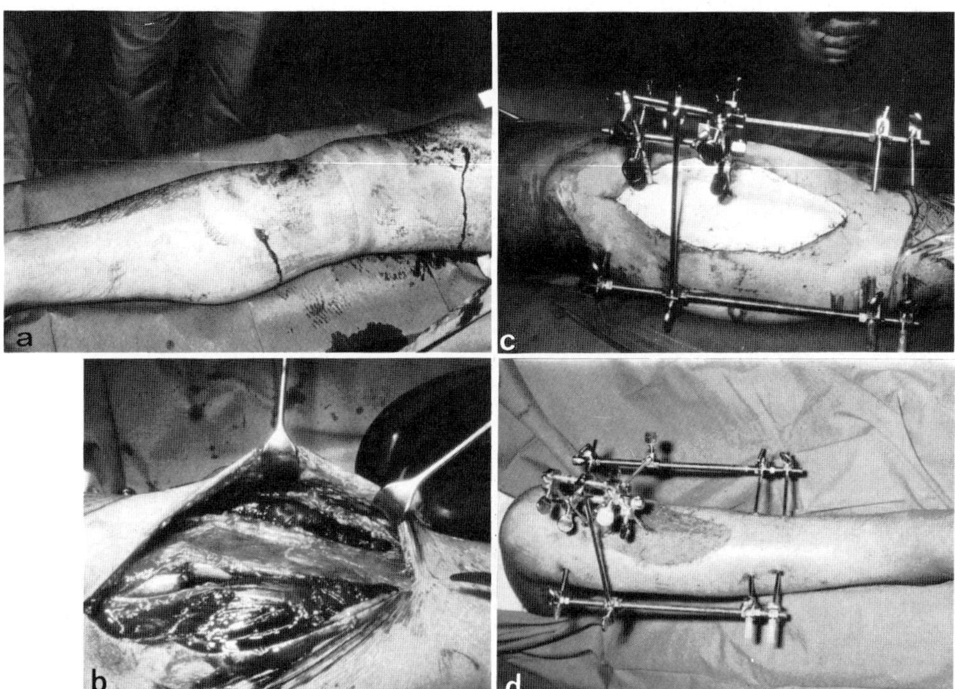

Fig. 13a–d. An 18-year-old motorcyclist sustained an open fracture of the right femoral shaft and proximal tibia. He was in profound shock when admitted 1 hour postinjury. Two puncture wounds were visible on the right lower leg, which was severely swollen. The muscles about the calf and remainder of the lower leg were very tense, firm and painful. Pedal pulses were absent, but evidence of capillary flow was noted (**a**). A diagnosis of compartment syndrome was made, and, dispensing with angiography, immediate decompression was carried out. Inspection of the wounds revealed an extensive subcutaneous avulsion around the anterior puncture wound, and so a midline longitudinal incision was utilized (**a**). Marked pathologic changes in the muscles were immediately apparent. When the posterior compartment was opened, a mushroom-like bulge of muscle protruded through the incision (**b**). Following debridement, the tibial fracture was stabilized by external fixation, and the femoral fracture was plated. The wound was left open, and synthetic skin was sutured into the defect. The fracture was covered with periosteum (**c**). Seven days later the defect was covered with a meshed graft, and uneventful healing ensured (**d**). The injury is classified as Fr. O III on the basis of soft tissue lesions

Delayed Wound Closure

Delayed wound closure is the most common method of managing wounds associated with open fractures.

a) Secondary suture. After posttraumatic edema has passed, the decrease in soft tissue tension often makes it easy to obtain tension-free closure of a primary wound or secondary

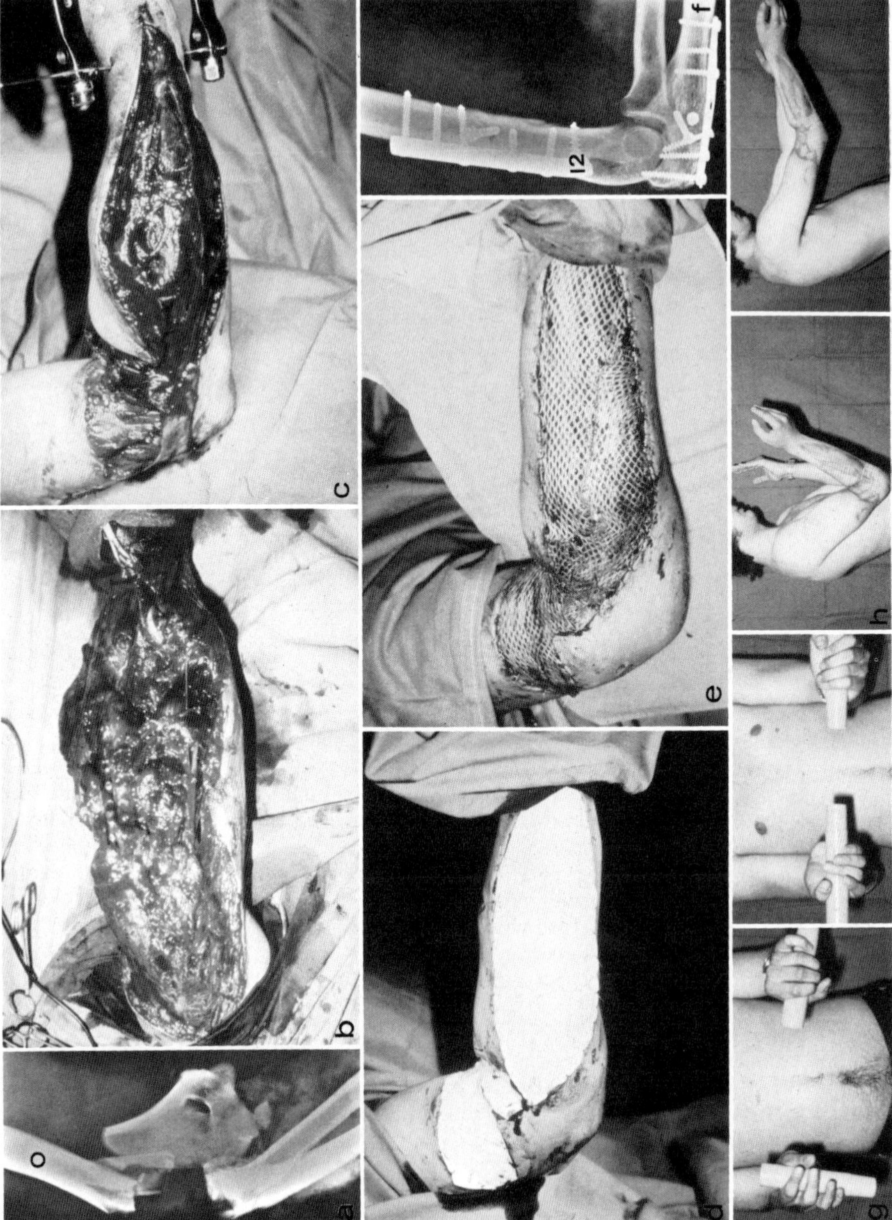

Fig. 14a–h. Grade III open fractures of the upper extremity sustained during a motorcycle accident: humeral shaft fracture and fracture-dislocation of the elbow with extensive muscle damage on the dorsal aspect of the forearm "floating elbow" (**a**, **b**). Following debridement and internal fixation, all wounds were left open (**c**), covered first with synthetic skin (**d**), and then secondarily covered with meshed grafts (**e**). The fractures healed nicely, as seen in the 12-week roentgenograms (**f**). Mobility is acceptable in view of the severity of the soft-tissue and osseous injury (**g**, **h**)

incision (Fig. 17). Since we have been using the secondary suture, we have noticed a markedly lower incidence of soft tissue necrosis.

b) Split-thickness skin grafts. This type of grafting should not be done primarily. It is better to wait until posttraumatic edema has cleared and a granulating surface has formed. Four to ten days later, when the defect has decreased in size, it can be readily closed with a meshed split-thickness skin graft (Figs. 15, 16). A second look may be taken at this time. The wound should be kept moist with saline or povidone-iodine solution until closure is effected.

The foregoing techniques of soft tissue coverage are inadequate if there is an associated periosteal defect with exposure of the bone. In this situation, one of the following techniques must be selected. Because the bone tends to dry out quickly and become increas-

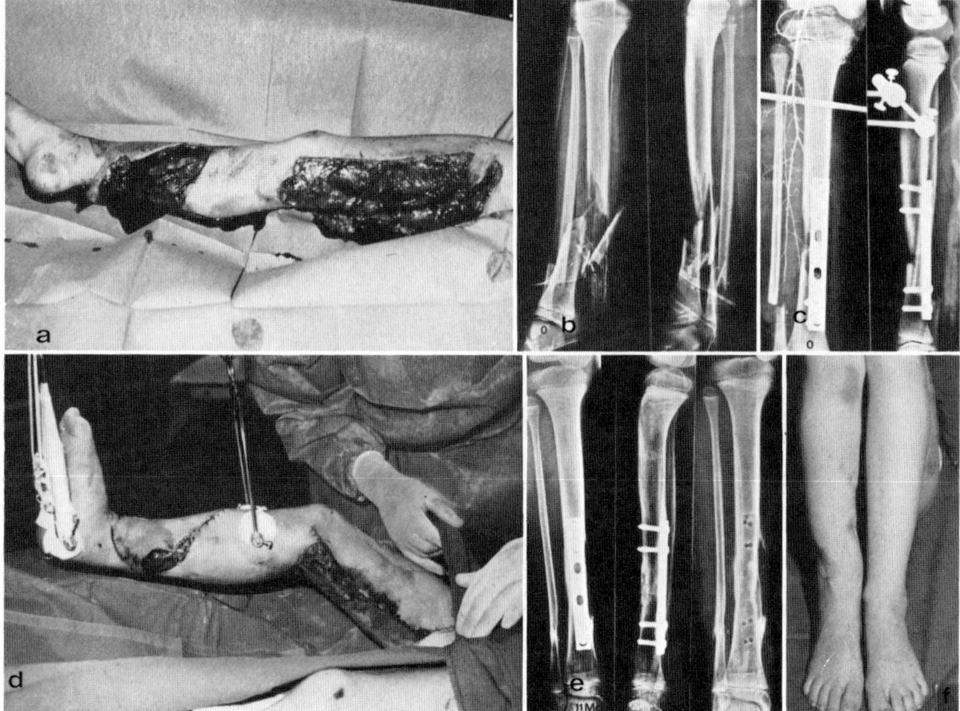

Fig. 15a–f. Grade III open tibial fracture with bone loss, damage to the posterior tibial artery and vein, and a large soft tissue wound on the medial side of the thigh (**a**, **b**). Following debridement, the tibia was stably plated on its posterior aspect. Primary bone grafting was not carried out (**c**). The wounds were left partially open. No significant soft tissue necrosis occurred despite the impairment of blood flow to the traumatic skin flaps. The extremity was suspended by means of two Steinmann pins (**d**). Secondary bone grafting and split-thickness skin grafting were carried out, and uncomplicated consolidation of the fracture followed (**e**). There is no loss of motion in the knee and ankle joints, and the condition of the soft tissue is good (**f**)

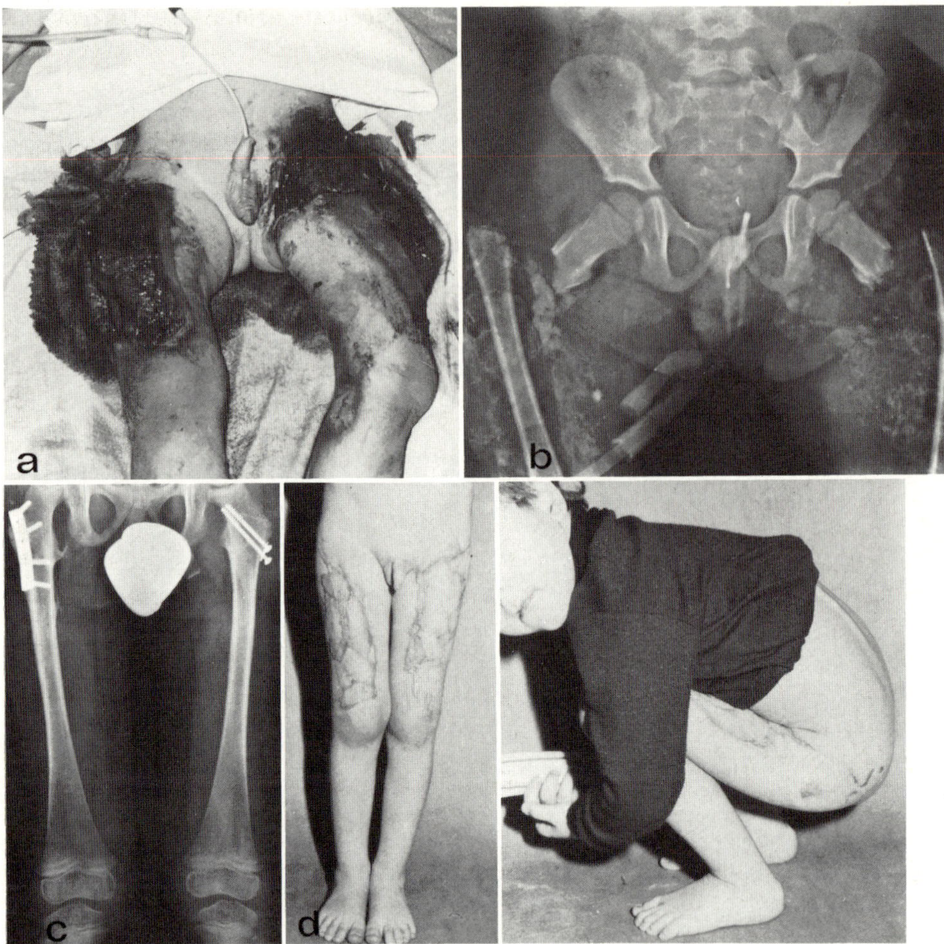

Fig. 16a–d. A 6-year-old boy was struck in the pelvis and femora by a dredger bucket while in a sand pit, sustaining widely open, heavily contaminated subtrochanteric fractures of both femora (**a**). Roentgenograms disclosed large amounts of foreign material in the soft tissues of the pelvis and femora. The sizable displacement attests to the very severe degree of soft tissue damage (**b**). The injury was managed in standard fashion by debridement, stable internal fixation with a minimum of implant material, and delayed closure with split-thickness skin grafts. Union is evident in the 4-month roentgenograms (**c**), at which time motion in all joints is unrestricted (**d**)

ingly compromised in its blood supply, the more arduous techniques of soft tissue reconstruction should be done either primarily or within 3–8 days after the injury.

c) Pedicle skin flaps. Pedicle skin flaps, such as rotation flaps and cross-leg flaps, are excellent for providing coverage in the face of full-thickness soft tissue loss.

d) Pedicle muscle flaps or myocutaneous flaps. This type of soft tissue reconstruction has proved especially useful for soft tissue defects of the lower leg (Fig. 17). The technique is described later.

e) Free tissue transfer with microvascular anastomosis. This technique is becoming increasingly important, but not as a primary measure.

5. Antibiotics and Postoperative Care

The problems connected with the use of prophylactic and therapeutic antibiotics and with postoperative care are discussed elsewhere in this volume.

Conclusions

The results of open fracture treatment are based largely on the accurate assessment and management of soft tissue injuries. The main principles in the treatment of open fractures may be summarized as follows:

1. Sterile bandaging, alignment and splinting of the open fracture at the accident scene are effective in preventing wound infection and additional soft tissue damage.
2. Preparations for surgery, wound debridement and irrigation must be carried out with painstaking care. Debridement includes the excision of all avascular and grossly dirty skin, bone and muscle.
3. The primary, stable operative fixation of the fracture creates optimum conditions for undisturbed osseous and soft tissue healing.
4. The wound must be closed without tension. In most cases the wound is left open and covered with synthetic skin.
   Delayed closure is done with a suture, split-thickness skin graft, pedicle flaps or free tissue transfer with microvascular anastomosis.
5. Close postoperative supervision is mandatory for the prevention of serious complications. At the first signs of complications, the patient is returned to OR for a second look and redebridement.

The treatment of open fractures requires a high level of knowledge and experience on the part of the attending surgeon with regard to the principles of wound care and fracture management.

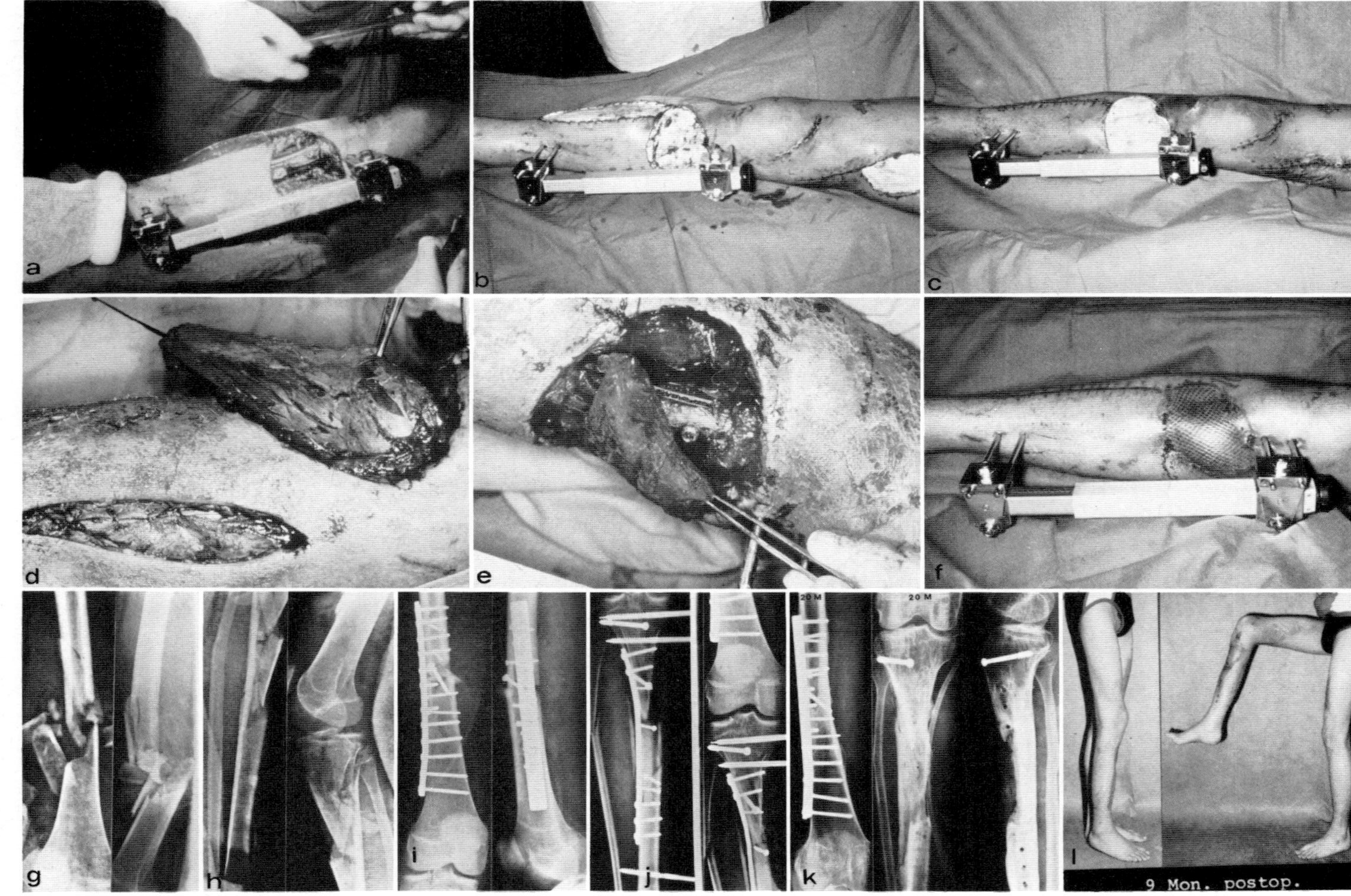
20 M
20 M
9 Mon. postop.

◄ **Fig. 17a–l.** A 19-year-old motorcyclist sustained grade III open fractures of the right femoral and tibial shaft (**g**, **h**). The femoral fracture was plated (**i**), and lateral plating of the tibia was supplemented by medial external fixation with a Wagner device. A large medial bone defect remained (**j**). Soft tissue coverage was also lacking over this defect (**a**). The wounds of the upper and lower leg were partially closed, and synthetic skin was sutured into the remaining skin defects (**b**). After posttraumatic edema had subsided, the wounds were closed by secondary suture. Synthetic skin was again used to cover the soft-tissue and osseous defect on the medial tibia (**c**). Eight days postinjury a muscle flap was mobilized from the medial gastrocnemius (**d**) and swung over the defect (**e**). A split-thickness meshed skin graft was applied over the muscle (**f**). The soft tissues healed without complications. Secondary bone grafting was followed by good bony union, as seen in the 20-month films (**k**). Condition of soft tissues and knee mobility 9 months after operation (**l**)

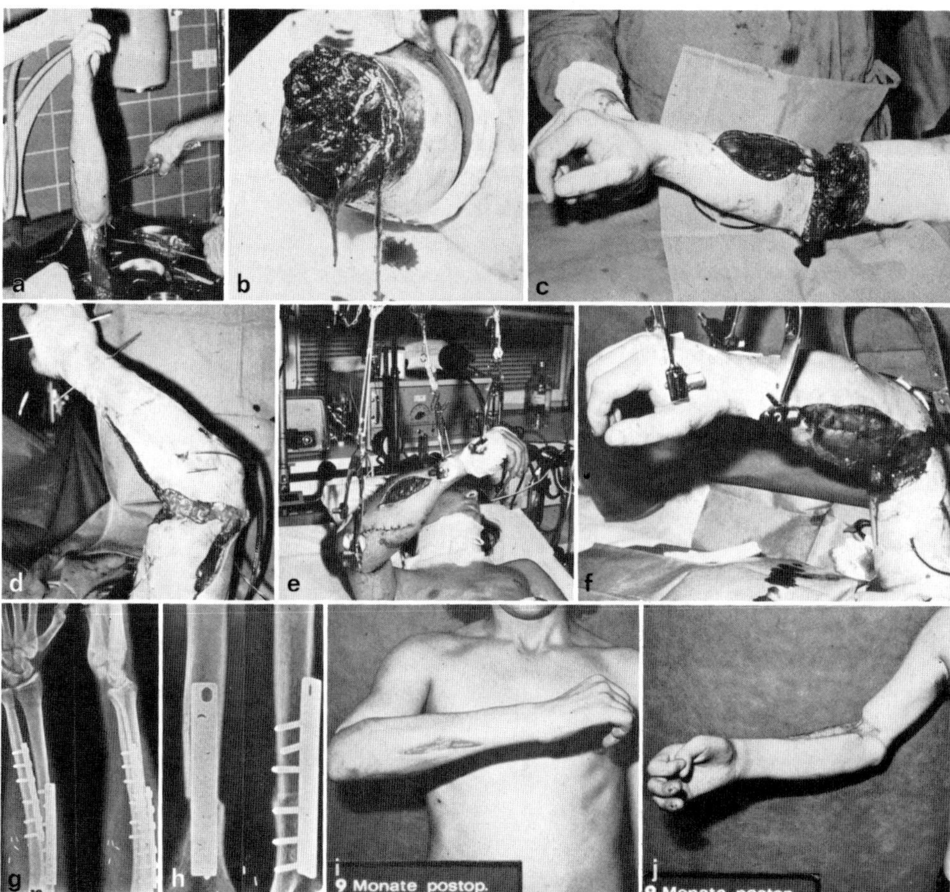

Fig. 18a–j. A 22-year-old man was involved in a high-speed auto accident, sustaining an above-elbow avulsion of the right arm. There was also a closed forearm fracture in the avulsed member (**a**). Amputation stump (**b**). Immediate replantation was carried out. Following wound debridement, a shortening osteotomy was performed on the humerus and stabilized with a plate. The ruptured vessels were repaired, the forearm fracture was plated, and torn muscles and nerves were sutured. Skin closure was minimal, and all fasciae were incised, especially in the forearm (**c**, **d**). Positioning of the extremity in ICU (**e**, **f**). 12-week roentgenograms show uncomplicated fracture union (**g**, **h**). Range of arm motion 9 months postoperatively (**i**, **j**); after that time the whereabouts of the patient, a drug user, could not be ascertained

References

1. Allgöwer M (1971) Weichteilprobleme und Infektionsrisiko der Osteosynthese. Arch Chir 329:1128
2. Billroth T (1866) Die allgemeine und chirurgische Pathologie und Therapie in 50 Vorlesungen. Reimer, Berlin
3. Burri C (1974) Posttraumatische Osteitis. Huber, Bern Stuttgart Wien
4. Heppenstall RB (1980) Fracture Treatment and Healing. Saunders, Philadelphia London Toronto
5. Matter P (1970) Grundsätzliche Indikationsfehler bei offenen Frakturen. Arch Chir 327:858
6. Rittmann WW, Pusterla C, Matter P (1969) Früh- und Spätinfektionen bei offenen Frakturen. Helv Chir Acta 36:537
7. Rittmann WW, Matter P (1977) Die offene Fraktur. Huber, Bern Stuttgart Wien
8. Rojczyk M (1981) Keimbesiedlung und Keimverhalten bei offenen Frakturen. Unfallheilkunde 84:458
9. Rojczyk M (1981) Anwendungsmöglichkeiten von Epigard bei offenen Frakturen. In: Weller S, Weiss K, Hopf KH (Hrsg) Möglichkeiten der temporären Wunddeckung. Gödecke AG, Abt Meditechnika, Freiburg
10. Rojczyk M, Tscherne H (1982) Bedeutung der praeklinischen Versorgung bei offenen Frakturen. Unfallheilkunde 85:72
11. Tscherne H, Magerl F, Fleischl P (1967) Die Marknagelung frischer offener und geschlossener Unterschenkelfrakturen. Langenbecks Arch Chir 317:209
12. Tscherne H (1969) Operative Frakturbehandlung. Langenbecks Arch Chir 317:209
13. Tscherne H (1972) Die Weichteilversorgung bei offenen Frakturen. Schriftenr Unfallmed Tag Landesverb Gewerbl Berufsgen 14:17
14. Tscherne H (1982) Primäre Behandlung der Oberarmschaftfrakturen. Langenbecks Arch Chir 332:379
15. Tscherne H, Schmit-Neuerburg KP (1974) Therapeutische Indikationen bei Frakturen langer Röhrenknochen. In: Heberer G, Hegemann G (Hrsg) Indikation zur Operation. Springer, Berlin Heidelberg New York
16. Tscherne H, Oestern HJ (1974) Konservative oder operative Frakturbehandlung bei kompletter Unterarmfraktur. Akt Traumatol 4:85
17. Tscherne H, Brüggemann H (1974) Die sekundäre Versorgung der Weichteile bei offenen Frakturen. In: Naumann HH, Kartenbauer ER (Hrsg) Plastisch-chirurgische Maßnahmen nach frischen Verletzungen. Thieme, Stuttgart
18. Tscherne H (1975) Die Behandlung der offenen Frakturen. 10. Unfallseminar, Hannover
19. Tscherne H (1976) Oberarm. In: Baumgartl F, Kremer K, Schreiber HW (Hrsg) Spezielle Chirurgie für die Praxis, Bd III/1. Thieme, Stuttgart
20. Tscherne H, Brüggemann H (1976) Die Weichteilbehandlung bei Osteosynthesen, insbesondere bei offenen Frakturen. Unfallheilkunde 79:467
21. Tscherne H, Oestern HJ (1976) Unterarmschaftbrüche. Schriftenr Unfallmed Tag Landesverb Gewerbl Berufsgen 27:199
22. Tscherne H (1977) Offene kindliche Frakturen. Z Kinderchir 22:61
23. Tscherne H (1978) Technik und Ergebnisse der Plattenosteosynthese am Unterarmschaft. Unfallheilkunde 81:332
24. Tscherne H (1981) Treatment of Fractures with Concomitant Soft Tissue Injuries. Instructional Course Lecture. XV World Congr of SICOT, Rio de Janeiro, Brasil
25. Volkmann R (1878) Die Behandlung der complizierten Fracturen. Zentralbl Chir 5: 649
26. Weller S, Weiss K, Hopf KH (1980) Möglichkeiten der temporären Wunddeckung. Gödecke AG, Abt Meditechnika, Freiburg

Results of the Treatment of Open Fractures, Aspects of Antibiotic Therapy

M. Rojczyk

1. Introduction

Open fractures have for a long time lost the stigma of being a lethal injury. Nevertheless, considering the fact that, in our practice, some 52% of patients with open fractures have sustained multiple injuries, these patients still run a relatively high risk of death or disability. At 8.3%, the mortality rate among open-fracture patients is still significant.

Table 1 shows the major causes of death in patients with open fractures, listed in order of frequency and chronology. Shock sequelae are generally fatal within the first 48 hours. The consequences of serious head injury tend to be fatal within the first week. "Trauma lung" or respiratory distress syndrome is mainly important in elderly patients and is most pronounced during the second week. Nowadays, this cause of death has been virtually eliminated owing to improvements in the management of multiple trauma patients and is being replaced by sepsis during the 2nd through 4th week – also a shock sequela marked by multiple organ failure. The open fracture itself is of no consequence in septic deaths. Pneumonia, pulmonary embolism, gastrointestinal bleeding and other complications may still threaten the life of elderly patients several weeks after the trauma.

Table 1. Causes of death in 49 patients with 64 open fractures

Schock sequelae	20 deaths
Head injury	15 deaths
Trauma lung/respiratory distress	9 deaths
Sepsis	4 deaths
Pneunomia	1 death

2. Clinical Material and Results

At the Hannover Medical School, 678 open fractures were treated during the period from 1972 to 1980. The localizations of the fractures are shown schematically in Fig. 1. It is seen that 80% of all fractures occurred in the lower extremity, with 50% affecting the tibia. Open fractures of the hand, foot, chest, pelvis and skull were excluded from the review.

Table 2 shows the severity of the associated soft tissue injury. Fifty-seven vascular injuries were recorded.

Over 50% of all the open fractures were stabilized by plate fixation (Table 3). Intramedullary nailing (9%) was utilized mainly for grade I open fractures, as were most of the 15% of fractures managed primarily by nonoperative means. The most common indication

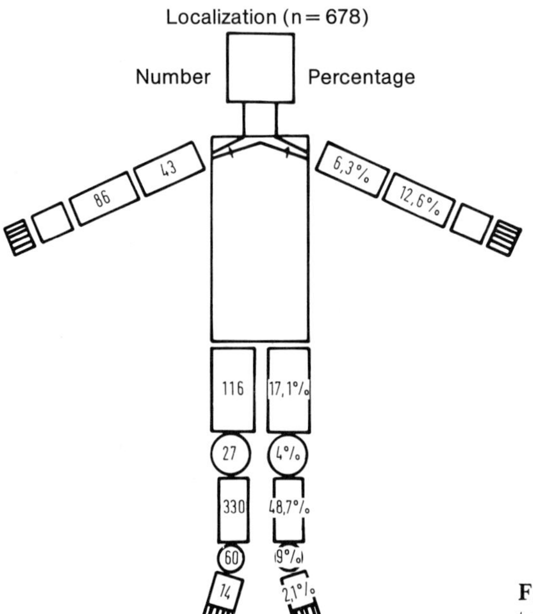

Fig. 1. Localization of 678 open fractures treated from 1972 to 1980

Table 2. Severity of soft tissue trauma associated with 678 open fractures

Fr. O I	208	(30.7%)
Fr. O II	276	(40.7%)
Fr. O III	169	(25.0%)
Fr. O IV	25	(3.7%)
Vascular injuries	57	(8.4%)

Table 3. Modality of treatment for 678 open fractures

Primary conservative	104	(15.3%)
Intramedullary nailing	60	(8.9%)
Plate fixation	347	(51.2%)
External fixation	37	(5.4%)
Other fixation	104	(15.3%)
Primary amputation	29	(4.3%)
Secondary amputation	15	(2.2%)

for external fixation was a very severe degree of soft tissue damage associated with tibial fractures. "Other fixation" includes tension banding, screw fixation and Kirschner wire fixation. Besides 29 primary amputations, there were 15 secondary amputations performed a short time after the first operation, due mainly to ischemic complications.

Of 57 diagnosed concomitant vascular injuries, 25 were repaired by suture or vein graft. The remainder were ligated, or the extremity was amputated primarily (Table 4).

Table 4. Treatment of 57 vascular injuries

Primary amputation/ligation	32	(56.1%)
Repair/reconstruction	25	(43.9%)

The overall incidence of osseous infections in the patient population, excluding amputees and fatalities, is 5.6% (Table 5). In all 32 cases, complete osseous healing could be achieved. Eighty percent of the open fractures had gone on to complete union by 4 months post-injury, and 95% by 8 months. All but 5 of the infected pseudarthroses had healed completely within a year (Table 6).

Table 5. Osseous infections in 570 open fractures

Total number	32	(5.6%)
Fr. O I	7	(3.7%)
Fr. O II	6	(2.4%)
Fr. O III	19	(10.6%)

Table 6. Fracture healing times for 570 open fractures

4 months	493	(79.7%)
4–8 months	84	(14.6%)
8–12 months	28	(4.8%)
12 months	5	(0.9%)

Fracture healing times were determined from roentgenograms and hospital records. At present, detailed follow-up results are available for a series of 220 open fractures admitted between 1972 and 1975 (Table 7). The localization and severity of the soft tissue trauma correspond roughly to that of the total patient population.

Table 7. Functional results in a review of 220 open fractures (1972–1975)

Good	181	(82.3%)
Fair	32	(14.5%)
Poor	7	(3.2%)

The results of treatment were rated according to the following criteria:

Good: Unrestricted joint motion, axial deformity up to 5°, no pain on weight bearing, limp-free gait.

Fair: Motion restricted up to 25% in one adjacent joint, axial deformity up to 5°, pain on prolonged weight bearing, slight limp.

Poor: Motion restricted more than 25% in one adjacent joint, axial deformity greater than 5°, pain on weight bearing, marked limp, walking aids required.

On the basis of this criteria, 82.3% of the follow-up cases were rated as good, 14.5% as fair, and 3.2% as poor. The percentage of poor results is significantly lower than the rate of osseous infections. Cases with primary and secondary amputations were excluded from the review.

Preventive Antibiotics

The term "prophylactic antibiotics" is appropriate only for antibiotics which are administered in large doses for a short time during aseptic operations. It is better to use the term "preventive antibiotics" when dealing with open fractures, in which wound contamination is a virtual certainty.

The value of preventive antibiotics remains controversial. At one time, we rejected the use of antibiotics in the treatment of open fractures, except as a nonabsorbable additive to the irrigating solution. However, when studies in the U.S. (Patzakis 1974) pointed to a significant decline of infection rates in patients treated with antibiotics, we were prompted to test the validity of our policy on the basis of a prospective study.

The material consisted of a closed series of 199 open fractures admitted during the period from June, 1977, to December, 1979. We divided the patients into two groups as follows: Patients admitted on odd-numbered days were started preoperatively on cephazolin at a dose of 1 g q.i.d. This was maintained for at least 5 days. Intensive-care patients and patients on respirators were occasionally switched to azlocillin at 5 g t.i.d.

Patients with open fractures who were admitted on even-numbered days did not receive antibiotics.

In the same population, regular smears were taken before, during and after surgery to monitor the level of bacterial contamination in the wounds (Rojczyk 1981).

On the 199 open fractures that were treated, 111 were in the group with antibiotics and 88 in the group without antibiotics (Tables 8 and 9). Taking the total prevalence of soft tissue infections and osseous infections together, we found a 7.2% infection rate in the group with antibiotics, as opposed to a 13.8% infection rate in the group without antibiotics. Although this difference is not statistically significant in the chi-square test, we felt that it nevertheless had valid implications with regard to the value of preventive antibiotic therapy.

Since 1980, therefore, preventive antibiotics are routinely administered to all of our open-fracture patients for a period of 24 to 48 hours. Table 10 shows the infection rate of the patient population for 1980. At 7.9%, this rate is practically identical to that of the antibiotic group in the previous study. In contrast to earlier investigations (Patzakis 1974),

Table 8. Infection rates for 111 open fractures treated with antibiotics

Soft tissue infection	5	(4.5%)
Ossseous infection	3	(2.7%)
Total	8	(7.2%)

Table 9. Infection rates for 88 open fractures treated without antibiotics

Soft tissue infection	7	(8.0%)
Osseous infection	5	(5.8%)
Total	12	(13.8%)

the infection rate did not rise again after termination of the study, but remained at a low level.

The primary wound smear taken at regular intervals during the study were found to contain mostly saprophytic organisms such as micrococci, diphtheroids, saprophytic rods, etc. This is precisely what one would expect in wounds contaminated with soil and road dirt. Pathogenic organisms were demonstrated in only 20 cases. Of these, 8 (40%) developed a wound infection (soft-tissue or osseous). In 179 cases with predominantly saprophytic organisms, 12 wound infections (6.4%) occurred (Table 11). Thus, in open fractures that were primarily contaminated with pathogenic organisms, the risk of infection was drastically increased.

We have drawn the following additional therapeutic conclusions from these findings: All patients with open fractures receive cephazolin, 2 g t.i.d., for 24–48 hours, starting before their operation. After that period the result of the primary wound smear is obtained by telephone. If pathogenic organisms have been found, treatment with a specific antibiotic selected on the basis of sensitivity tests is instituted and maintained for at least 5 days.

Table 10. Infection rates for 88 open fractures in 1980

Soft tissue infection	3	(3.4%)
Osseous infection	4	(4.5%)
Total	7	(7.9%)

Table 11. Demonstration of pathogenetic organisms in the primary wound smear

Positive: 20	Negative: 179
Infection rate:	
8 (40.0%)	12 (6.7%)

In this way, broad-spectrum, nonspecific antibiotics with their undesired effects can be largely avoided. When wound closure is deferred, antibiotics should be continued until definitive wound coverage is obtained.

Despite the positive aspects of antibiotic therapy, it should be emphasized that the administration of antibiotics is adjunctive only and is useful only in conjunction with appropriate surgical treatment.

References

1. Gustilo RB (1979) Use of antimicrobials in the management of open fractures. Arch Surg 114:805
2. Hierholzer G, Lob G (1978) Antibioticatherapie in der Unfallchirurgie. Unfallheilkd 81:64
3. Patzakis HJ, Harvey JP, Yvler D (1974) The role of antibiotics in the management of open fractures. J Bone Joint Surg 56:532
4. Rojczyk M (1981) Keimbesiedlung und Keimverhalten bei offenen Frakturen. Unfallheilkd 84:458
5. Stolle D, Naumann P, Kremer K, Loose DA (1980) Antibiotica-Prophylaxe in der Traumatologie. Hefte Unfallheilkd 143

The Treatment of Closed Fractures with Soft Tissue Injuries

H. Tscherne and M. Rojczyk

1. Introduction

Increasingly, closed fractures with associated soft tissue injuries are presenting the attending physician with difficult decisions in terms of diagnosis and management (Tscherne, Brüggemann 1976; Weiss et al. 1978). The soft tissue trauma is usually more difficult to evaluate than in open fractures, often causing the surgeon to underestimate the true extent of the damage. A full-thickness skin contusion is a more serious injury than the simple skin perforation characteristic of open fractures. Skin necrosis leading to secondary infection is a typical complication of the closed injury. Even in the absence of full-thickness necrosis, the contusion can disrupt the integrity of the cutaneous barrier, rendering it permeable to bacteria.

A unique feature of these injuries is that the primary damage can become greatly exacerbated as a result of swelling and the associated pressure increase. The time factor is of critical importance, and *every closed fracture with soft tissue injury is a true surgical emergency.*

2. Preoperative Measures

The fractures should be reduced and immobilized in a pneumatic splint before moving the patient from the accident scene. Otherwise, the pressure exerted on soft tissues by the bone fragments is apt to cause additional injury, ischemia or even compounding before definitive care can be given. Upon arrival at the hospital, the injured extremity is examined for adequacy of blood flow and sensory and motor function, the soft tissues are closely inspected and palpated (especially for signs of compartment syndrome), and roentgenograms are obtained before further treatment is decided upon.

3. Treatment of Fractures with Grade I or II Soft Tissue Injuries

Fractures with grade I or II soft tissue injuries do not necessarily require surgical treatment. However, it is important to watch for signs of circulatory impairment or sensory and motor deficits so that a developing compartment syndrome will be promptly recognized. Analgesics should be used advisedly. *Increasing pain following reduction, pain on muscle stretching, progressive swelling, tension bullae and neurovascular symptoms are urgent warning signals.*

In the unconscious patient, the continuous instrumental monitoring of compartmental pressures is recommended in areas where the syndrome is likely to develop.

If, from the nature of the fracture, it is felt that operative treatment is indicated, *the operation should be undertaken as soon as possible,* preferably within the first 6–8 hours. Even deep abrasions are not a contraindication to primary operative stabilization. Indeed, the timing of surgery in the presence of abrasions or circumscribed contusions is never more favorable than immediately following the injury. Regardless of the treatment method that is chosen, all abrasions should be cleansed by brushing and irrigating with povidone-iodine solution before surgery is performed or before a closed reduction is undertaken. Otherwise there will be an unacceptable risk of secondary infection.

An *impending perforation of the skin* over a fracture that cannot be reduced conservatively demands *immediate surgical intervention.* The typical example is an irreducible fracture-dislocation of the ankle joint with valgus displacement and pressure on the skin from the sharp edge of the fractured medial malleolus (Fig. 1).

The skin incision conform to the standard approaches for closed fractures (Fig. 2). It must be decided on a case-by-case basis whether it is best to circumvent skin contusions and deep abrasions, or to make the incisions through damaged areas. Remember: *Implants must always be covered by well-perfused tissue.* Under no circumstances should implants be placed beneath contused or endangered skin. Long skin incisions improve operative exposure while minimizing skin tension and retractor pressure on soft tissues.

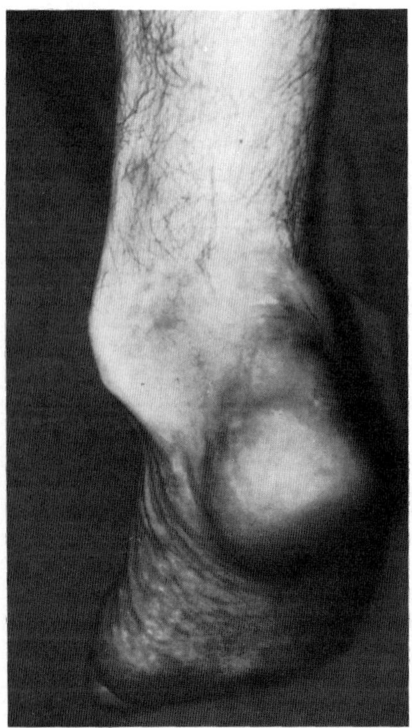

Fig. 1. Typical grade I soft tissue injury associated with a fracture-dislocation of the ankle joint. Immediate reduction and decompression of the soft tissues is indicated. Operative fixation, if necessary, should be undertaken without delay

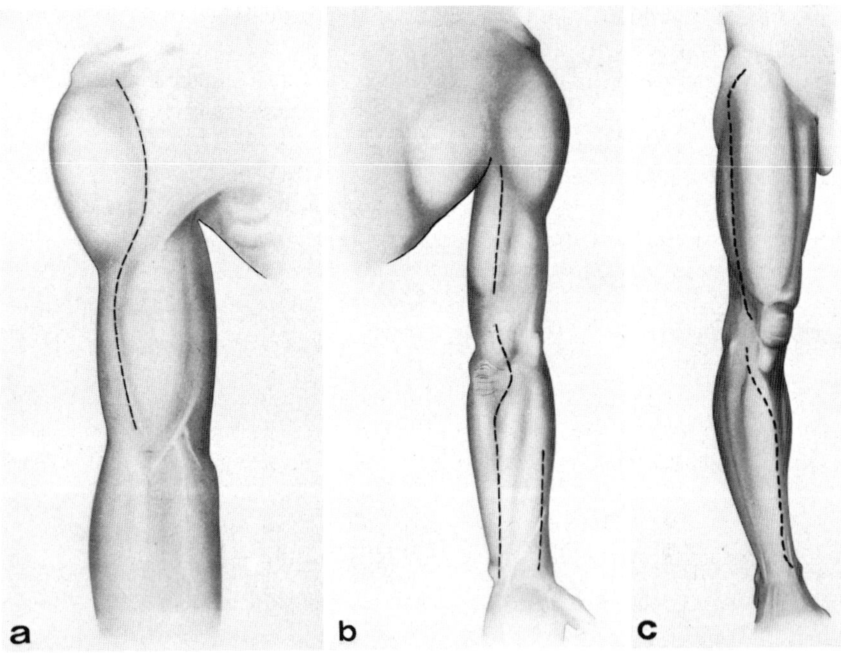

Fig. 2. Standard approaches for the operative treatment of closed fractures of the upper and lower extremity

4. Treatment of Fractures with Grade III Soft Tissue Injury

Unless managed operatively, nearly all fractures with grade III soft tissue injury will lead to a severe compartment syndrome (Fig. 3). Thus, to preserve the function of the extremity, *surgical treatment with decompression of the soft tissues* is urgently indicated.

When circulatory impairment is noted in the injured limb, differentiation between a *vascular injury* and *compartment syndrome* may prove difficult. If a diagnosis cannot be established by clinical methods or Doppler ultrasonography, angiograms should be obtained.

The operative technique corresponds to that for open fractures. After the skin is incised, the overlying fascia is divided at once so that a rapid decompression can be effected. A thorough debridement is just as important as a stable reduction of the fracture. Both stages of the operation are essential for avoiding further soft tissue necrosis and the secondary infection that very often follows. In the tibial region, external fixation is the method of stabilization in such cases. If the soft tissue damage extends beyond an adjacent joint, the external fixator can be applied in an articular transfixing configuration with little additional effort (Fig. 4).

Wound closure is governed by the same criteria outlined for open fractures. This means that, in most cases, the *skin incision is left open or is only partially closed.* Temporary coverage with synthetic skin followed by secondary closure with sutures is generally the method of choice.

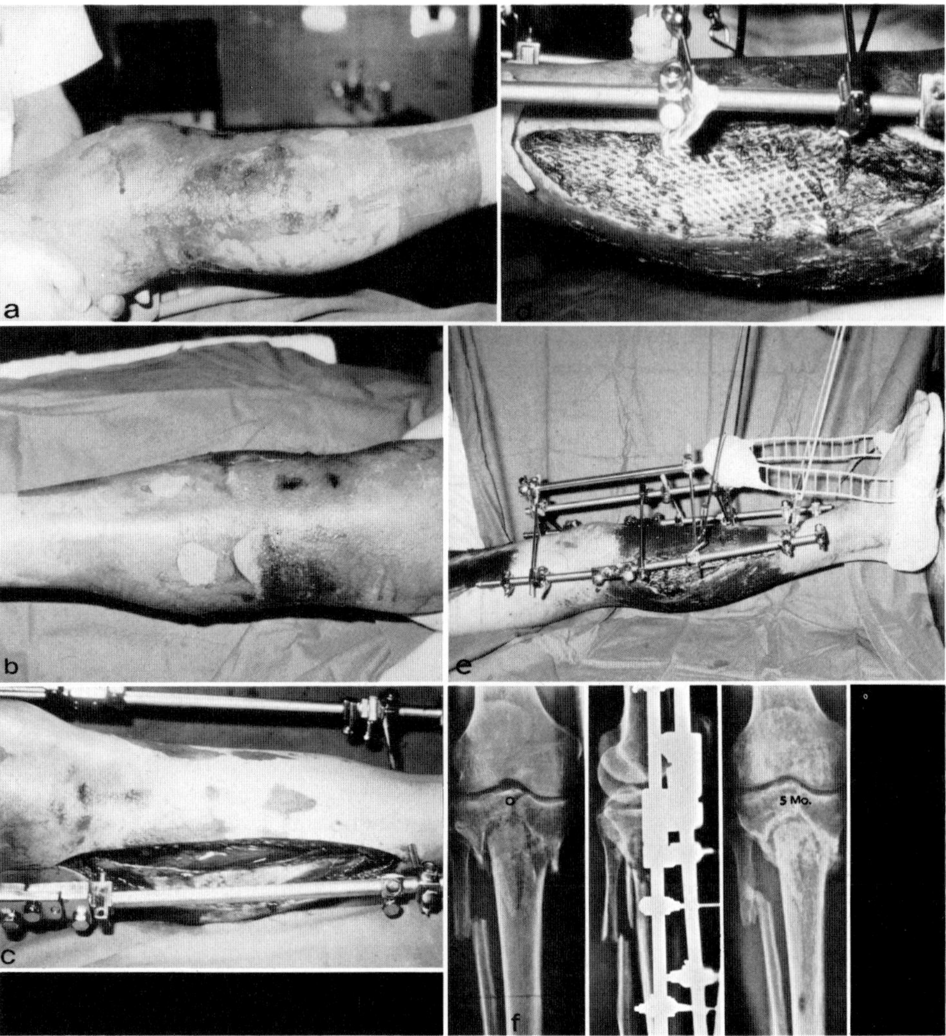

Fig. 3a–f. A 42-year-old bicyclist was struck by an automobile, sustaining a closed fracture of the upper tibia. He was transferred to our unit one day after the accident due to a progressive compartment syndrome. On admission, a grade III soft tissue injury was apparent: the soft tissues were greatly swollen, the skin was tense, isolated tension bullae were present, and discoloration from hematomas and contusions was evident on the anterior and posterior aspects of the limb. All muscle compartments were hard and tender to pressure (**a**, **b**). A closed reduction was carried out and stabilized by applying an external frame which crossed the knee joint. All four fascial compartments were incised. The wounds were left open (**c**) until covered secondarily with a meshed graft (**d**, **e**). The external frame was left in place for 4 weeks, followed by a short period of mobilization on a motion splint; therapy was completed in a plaster dressing (**f**)

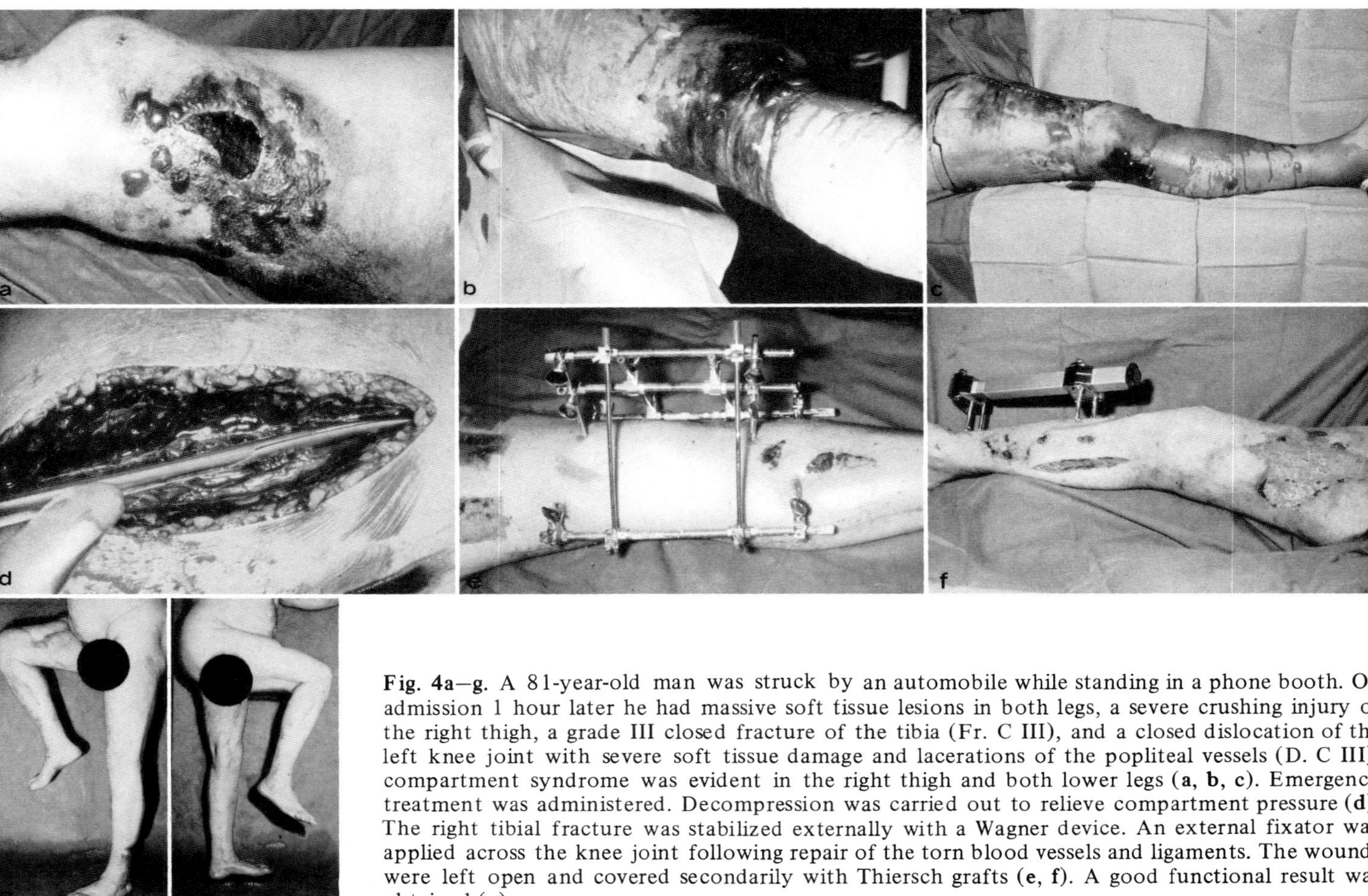

Fig. 4a–g. A 81-year-old man was struck by an automobile while standing in a phone booth. On admission 1 hour later he had massive soft tissue lesions in both legs, a severe crushing injury of the right thigh, a grade III closed fracture of the tibia (Fr. C III), and a closed dislocation of the left knee joint with severe soft tissue damage and lacerations of the popliteal vessels (D. C III); compartment syndrome was evident in the right thigh and both lower legs (**a**, **b**, **c**). Emergency treatment was administered. Decompression was carried out to relieve compartment pressure (**d**). The right tibial fracture was stabilized externally with a Wagner device. An external fixator was applied across the knee joint following repair of the torn blood vessels and ligaments. The wounds were left open and covered secondarily with Thiersch grafts (**e**, **f**). A good functional result was obtained (**g**)

Prophylactic antibiotics are administered as for open fractures. In the face of very severe trauma to soft tissues, it often is extremely difficult to judge the necessary extent of wound debridement within an emergency care setting. If there is doubt as to the viability of tissues, it is best to leave the tissues in place (especially muscle) and return the patient to the operating room for a second look and redebridement at a later time. In cases of massive soft tissue trauma, it is essential that skin incisions and fasciotomies be left open if the circulation is to improve. Synthetic skin should be changed at frequent intervals, usually

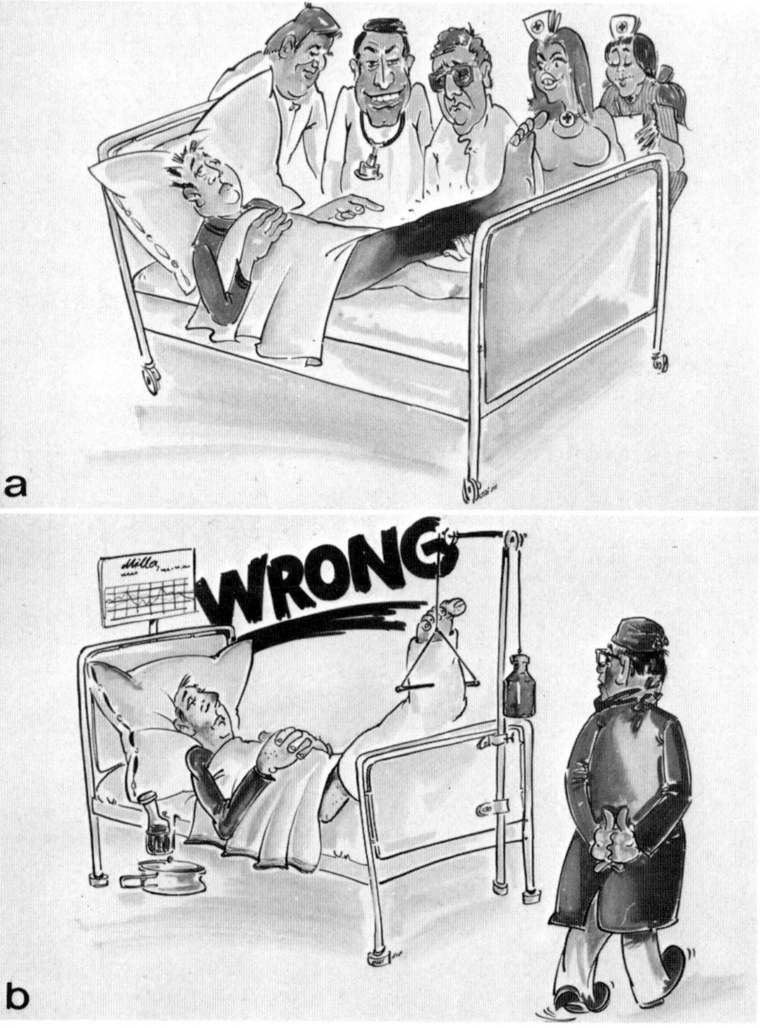

Fig. 5. Closed fractures with soft tissue injury can be difficult to diagnose and treat. With severe soft tissue trauma, a conservative approach is not advised (**a**, **b**). These injuries demand immediate surgical intervention

daily, to allow the inspection of soft tissues and the release of any hematomas that may have formed under the dressing. Open wound treatment may prove more favorable in some instances.

5. Conclusions

Closed fractures with soft tissue injuries often conceal serious lesions that are troublesome in terms of diagnosis, choice of treatment and surgical therapy. Ischemia and secondary infections leading to permanent functional deficits are typical complications. It is vital that the surgeon appreciate the significance of these injuries and recognize the need for urgent yet careful surgical intervention (Fig. 5).

References

Tscherne H, Brüggemann H (1976) Die Weichteilbehandlung bei Osteosynthesen, insbesondere bei offenen Frakturen. Unfallheilkd 79:467

Weiss H, Wissing H, Schmit-Neuerburg KP (1978) Komplikationsrate und Infektrisiko offener und geschlossener Unterschenkelbrüche mit Weichteilschaden. Akt Traumatol 8:329

The Operative Treatment of Tibial Shaft Fractures with Soft Tissue Injuries

L. Gotzen and N. Haas

1. Introduction

The tibial shaft fracture with associated soft tissue injury is an especially difficult therapeutic problem due to the severity of the trauma and the frequency of complications. Primary operative treatment with wound debridement and internal or external fixation creates biological and biomechanical conditions that are optimal in terms of osseous and soft tissue healing. Although this therapeutic concept has found widespread acceptance, the literature contains reports of high infection rates and numerous aseptic disturbances of fracture healing in cases where operative fixation has been utilized (e.g., Smith 1974; Ruedi et al. 1976; Weiss et al. 1978; Szyszkowitz et al. 1981).

Besides errors of indication, we believe that the high complication rates are due mainly to technical flaws which have adverse biological and biomechanical consequences. The advantages of operative fixation are realized only if the method chosen is appropriate for the given soft tissue conditions and fracture configuration, and the correct operative technique is employed (Müller, Allgöwer, Schneider, Willenegger 1977).

In the sections that follow, we shall give recommendations on indications, fixation methods and operative techniques. These recommendations are based upon insights derived first from a critical analysis of our own clinical material, and second from the results of our own clinical and experimental research as well as that of other authors.

But first we shall examine several aspects of the anatomy and traumatization of the lower leg that are relevant to an understanding of its pathophysiology and treatment.

2. Remarks on the Anatomy and Traumatization of the Lower Leg

Anatomy

The soft tissues of the lower leg are arranged asymmetrically about the tibia. The anterior border and medial surface of the tibia are subcutaneous, being covered throughout their extent by tense, adherent skin. No other bone has such a large area of skin contact (Lanz-Wachsmuth 1972). On its lateral aspect, the tibia is covered by the dorsal extensors, which form a thin pad over the anterolateral surface. The posterior surface is covered by the massive calf muscles, which are four times more powerful in their action than the dorsal extensors (Lanz-Wachsmuth 1972). As they descend toward the malleolar region, the muscles merge with their tendons, thereby decreasing the lateral and posterior soft-tissue coverage of the tibia distally and causing the fibula to become subcutaneous.

The tibia shows variations of geometry and strength in accordance with the varying loads imposed upon its individual portions. The bone has no predominant "tension side," although a posteriorally-directed bending moment is created by the arrangement of the musculature (Kimura 1974).

The tibia derives its blood supply from the nutrient artery, the metaphyseal arteries and the periosteal vessels (Fig. 1).

The nutrient artery, which arises from the posterior tibial artery, enters the medullary cavity of the tibia from the posterolateral aspect at the junction of the proximal and middle thirds, after first descending through a long, oblique canal, where it is highly vulnerable to injury. Upon piercing the bone, the artery divides into several ascending branches and one larger, central, descending vessel. These branches form the origin of the endosteal, centrifugal vascular network which supplies the tibial diaphysis. This network has numerous anastomoses with the metaphyseal arteries – a fact of some relevance to tibial nutrition in traumatic or operative injuries of the main vessel (Nelson et al. 1960; Crock 1967; Brooker 1971; Schweiberer et al. 1974; Eitel 1981).

The periosteal vessels, which arise mainly from the anterior tibial artery and encircle the tibia from its posterior and lateral sides in a roughly segmental fashion, supply only the outermost 10%–30% of the cortex under ordinary circumstances (Nelson et al. 1960; Rhinelander 1974; Macnab, de Haas 1974; Schweiberer et al. 1974). If the nutrient artery is lost (e.g., as a consequence of intramedullary nailing), then the periosteal arteries, together with extraosseous vessels from adjacent soft tissues, can contribute significantly to the centripetal nutrition of the cortex and thus to bone healing (Gothmann 1961; Danckwardt-Lilieström et al. 1970; Macnab, de Haas 1974; Hildebrandt 1979; Stürmer, Schuchardt 1980).

Venous return is accomplished partly via the accompanying veins of the medullary arteries and partly via the periosteal veins (Nelson et al. 1960; Trueta 1974).

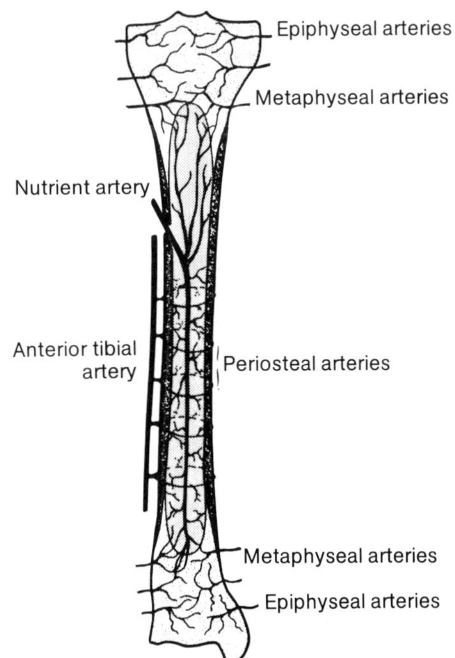

Fig. 1. Blood supply of the tibia

Traumatization

Vehicular accidents are by far the most common cause of tibial shaft fractures with soft tissue damage. Among our own patients, traffic accidents account for 90.5% of these injuries. The damage is mostly produced by high-energy deforming forces applied directly to the lower leg. Aided by the peculiar arrangement of the soft tissues in that region, the result is a massive traumatization of bone and soft tissue structures. Damage to soft tissue is based upon a combination of external and internal mechanisms (Fig. 2).

Lesions of the skin occur most frequently on the anteromedial aspect of the extremity (Fig. 3). The typical effects of direct violence to the skin and subcutis, such as contusions, perforations, lacerations and avulsions, are encountered in various combinations. In addition, there will always be some degree of muscle damage produced by the external trauma itself or secondarily by internal mechanisms.

Considerable swelling of the soft tissues may be expected in response to the trauma. This, together with internal hemorrhaging, leads to a sharp rise of tissue pressure, which in turn interferes with blood flow (Holden 1974, 1979).

Most tibial fractures are associated with marked displacement, widespread denudation of the fracture ends, separation of isolated fragments from their soft tissue attachments, and an extensive destruction of intramedullary vessels. Fractures with a butterfly fragment

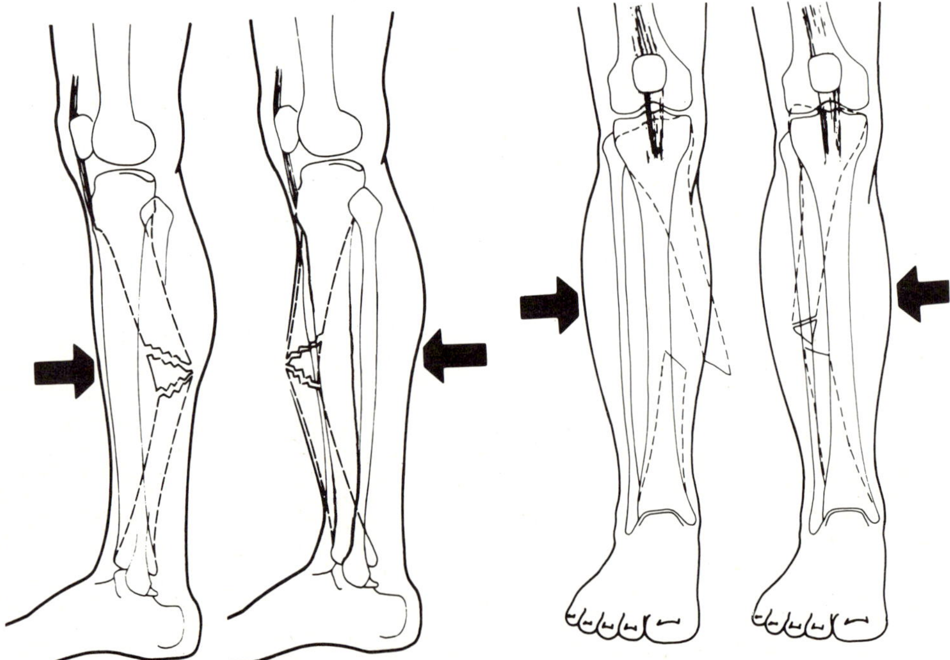

Fig. 2. Soft tissue damage from direct violence to the lower leg is the product of both external and internal mechanisms. Depending on the location and direction of the traumatizing force, the major soft tissue damage is caused primarily by the external trauma (impact) or secondarily by the internal trauma (fragment displacement)

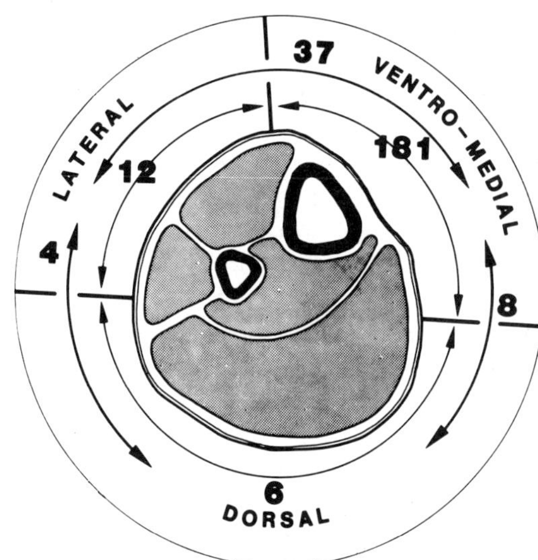

Fig. 3. Localization and frequency distribution of skin lesions in 260 open, operatively managed tibial fractures from the period 1976–1982

and comminuted fractures are the most common configurations. Segmental fractures and fractures with bone loss are seen in a fairly large percentage of cases (Fig. 4).

3. Indications Based upon Pathophysiologic Aspects

Soft tissue lesions and complex fracture configurations combined with significant impairment of tissue vascularity and viability are among the most difficult conditions to treat in the lower leg. The indications for the various methods of operative fixation, such as intra-

Triple fracture	Double fracture		Transverse fracture	Oblique fracture	Spiral fracture	Fracture with a butterfly fragment	Transverse – oblique fracture with short comminuted zone	Comminuted fracture	Fracture with bone loss
	6		3	7	2	4	4	18	–
2	7		21	22	6	49	25	44	7
	6		5	11	7	6	7	30	3
2	19		29	40	17	59	36	92	10

Fig. 4. Type and localization of 260 open tibial shaft fractures

medullary nailing, internal plating and external fixation, was well as the operative procedure itself must take special account of this unfavorable pathomorphologic situation.

Vascularity is the biological basis, and stability the biomechanical basis, of uncomplicated fracture healing (Rhinelander 1980). Both offer the best protection against infection. The greater the damage to the osseous vasculature, the greater the need for stability (Fig. 5).

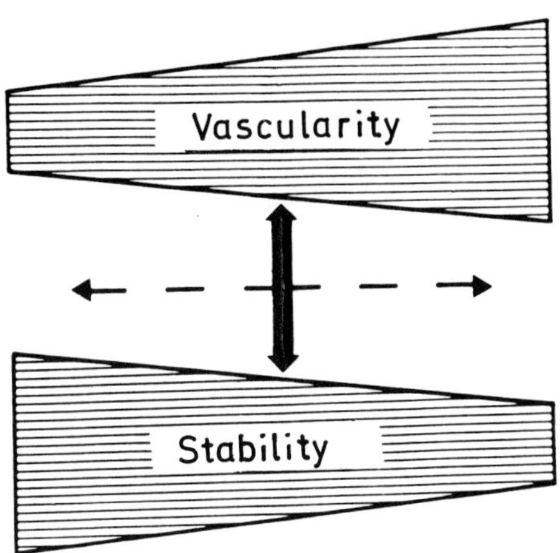

Fig. 5. Dependence of fracture healing on vascularity and stability

Stable fixation of the bone fragments ensures that the biological processes of revascularization and bone healing will be able to proceed without interference from disruptive mechanical influences. The viability of the fractured bone is determined essentially by the nature of the trauma that has been sustained. Care should be taken that fixation measures do not further compromise the blood supply to the bone, and that they promote revascularization.

Thus, biological conditions at the fracture site are the prime consideration in selecting a fixation method. It is true that a method should be used which is biomechanically suitable for a given fracture configuration, but only if it is acceptable from a biological standpoint. The adverse biological effects of the different fixation methods are of particular concern in this regard, for *biological considerations always take precedence over biomechanical requirements.* The selection of a stabilization method, then, must rely upon a critical assessment of the injury itself and of the various fixation techniques that are available. In particular, the following factors should be taken into account:

Fracture situation	Fixation method
↓	↓
Localization and nature of soft tissue trauma	**Biomechanical efficiency**
Localization and configuration of fracture	**Capacity for biological interference**
Fragment viability	
Bone quality	

There are overlaps of indication among the individual fixation methods, especially between internal plating and external fixation. The best rule to follow is: Use the method with which you are most familiar and which, given the circumstances, is associated with the lowest risks.

4. Wound Treatment and Operative Approach

The wound debridement that precedes operative fixation includes a sparing excision of the skin margins, meticulous cleansing of the wound, and the removal of all necrotic or devascularized tissue that is found in the fracture area.

Small cortical fragments devoid of soft tissue attachments should be discarded, but larger fragments may be replaced in some instances. Exposure of the fracture should be as atraumatic and limited as possible, should spare the soft tissues, and should not further jeopardize bone vitality.

A broader exposure is needed if plate fixation is contemplated. The location and size of the traumatic wound are taken into account when the incision is made (Schweiberer 1974; Tscherne, Brüggemann 1976; Rittmann, Matter 1977).

Longitudinal or oblique wounds on the anterior aspect of the lower leg (Fig. 6a, b) are incorporated into the standard lazy-S-shaped incision. With a transverse wound on the anterior side, a longitudinal incision can be made which includes the lateral or medial end of the wound, forming a pair of obtuse-angled skin flaps (Fig. 6c). With larger transverse wounds, we recommend making one or perhaps two separate longitudinal incisions, maintaining a distance of 4 cm from the site of the lesion (Fig. 6d, e). The standard incision may bypass the traumatic wound entirely if the latter is located more than 5 cm from the proposed line of incision (Fig. 6f).

5. Operative Fixation

In recent years there has been a marked change of attitudes toward the use of the various methods of operative fixation. In the belief that plate fixation carries an inordinately high risk of infection, more and more surgeons are turning to external fixation as a means of stabilizing fractures with severe soft tissue injuries (e.g., Karlström, Olerud 1977; Rittmann,

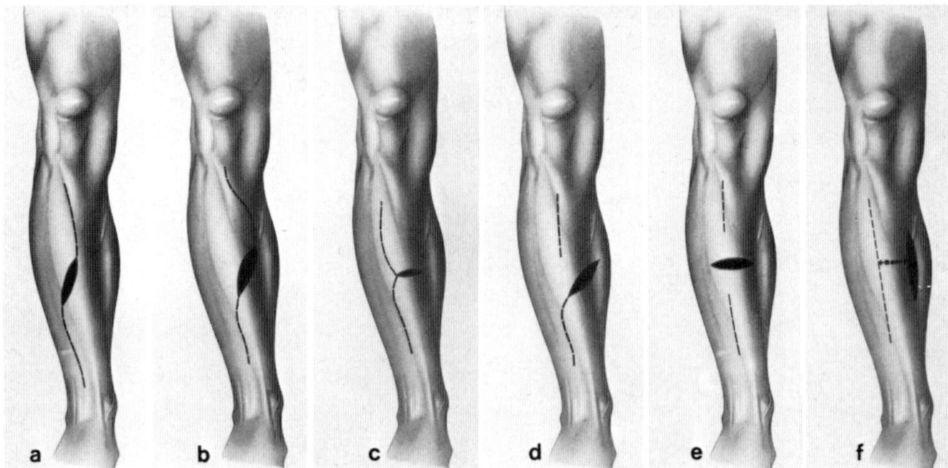

Fig. 6a–f. Various surgical approaches are available for internal plating of the tibia, depending on the location and size of the primary wound

Matter 1977; Knapp, Weller 1979; Lawyer 1979; Widenfalk et al. 1979; Burri et al. 1980; Szyskowitz et al. 1981; Klasen, Binnendyk 1982; Weller 1982). This is true in our own practice as well.

As Table 1 shows in the majority of fractures from the seven year period, plate fixation has been used mainly for fractures associated with moderately severe soft tissue injury. In grade III open fractures plate and external fixation was performed nearly with the same frequency.

For plate fixation an overall infection rate of 12.6% as opposed to 6.1% for external fixation was observed.

In 1982 external fixation has become our most commonly used modality for grade III soft tissue injuries and the preferred treatment for grade II open fractures. Among 45 open fractures there was only one infection. We believe that this low infection incidence is

Table 1. Degree of soft tissue lesions and fixation methods in 260 open, operatively managed tibial fractures from period 1976–1982; data for 1982 (n = 45) in parentheses

Soft tissue damage	I°		II°		III°		
Fixation methods							
Intramedullary nailing	25	(2)	8	(1)	–		33
Screw fixation	–		1		1		2
Plate fixation	17	(4)	92	(6)	51	(3)	160
External fixation			18	(9)	47	(20)	65

mainly due to the increased external fixation with biomechanically improved frame configurations in combination with an improved management of the soft tissue lesions.

Intramedullary Nailing

The intramedullary nail is a splinting implant whose tubular geometry gives it a high degree of mechanical strength. When loaded it does not bend and allows axial pressure to be transmitted to the fracture surfaces, producing a dynamic interfragmental compression which encourages periosteal callus formation.

On the other hand, of the three basic types of operative fixation, intramedullary nailing inflicts the greatest biological damage on the bone (Rhinelander 1974; Stürmer, Schuchardt 1980; Eitel 1981). Reaming of the medullary cavity and insertion of the nail destroy the intramedullary vascular system, and large portions of the cortex can become necrotic. Intramedullary revascularization is greatly hampered by contact between the nail and inner cortical wall and may take months to achieve.

If the bone ends have additionally been denuded of soft tissues over a large area as a result of periosteal and paraosseous damage, complete necrosis of the cortex will result. Bone healing is very seriously impaired, and the bone looses its resistance to infection.

Only if the soft tissue attachments of the bone ends are largely intact, enabling periosteal-extraosseous callus formation and centripetal cortical revascularization to occur (see Küntscher 1962), can the serious biological effects of intramedullary nailing be considered acceptable. Thus, given a suitable fracture localization and configuration, intramedullary nailing may be utilized for fractures with grade I or II closed soft tissue injury, grade I open fractures, and grade II open fractures in which the fragments are not significantly denuded of soft tissues (Fig. 7). Its use should not go beyond these indications.

With regard to technique, an effort should be made either to dispense with intramedullary reaming altogether or to keep the reaming to a minimum so that medullary trauma is reduced and a rapid regeneration of the medullary vascular system is encouraged. When closed nailing is done, the fracture hematoma and reaming debris should be flushed out via a separate incision in order to remove devitalized tissue and lower the internal pressure. If a compartment syndrome is anticipated or already present, the muscle compartments must be opened to effect a decompression (see Echtermeyer, Oestern).

Plate Fixation

The causes of the high complication rates of plate fixation are based essentially upon errors of indication, intraoperative tissue damage, deficiencies of soft tissue treatment and, above all, faulty technique. In other words, they are primarily iatrogenic in nature.

In a follow-up of 126 patients in whom we performed an open reduction and plate fixation, we recorded only 4 infections in 92 biomechanically sound fixations (4.3%), as opposed to 12 infections in 34 fixations with biomechanical deficiencies (35.2%). Aseptic healing complications requiring reoperation and malunion occurred only in cases where technical errors were made during application of the plates. The average consolidation time in stable fixations was 14.3 weeks. In fixations with instability-related complications, an

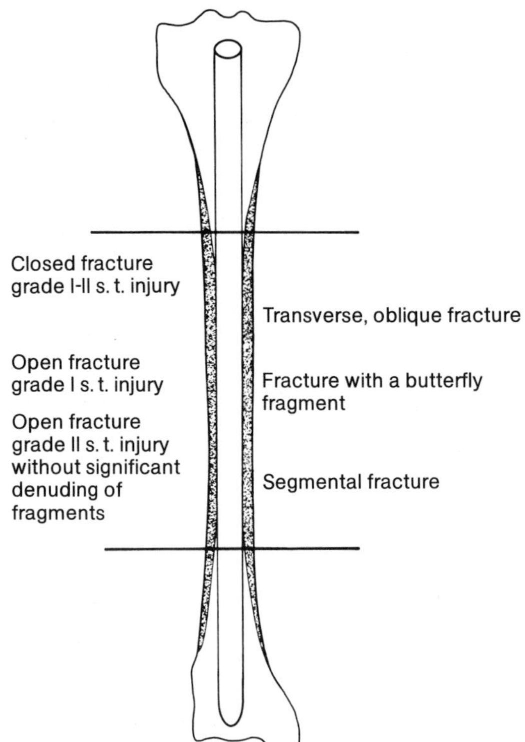

Fig. 7. Indications for intramedullary nailing in tibial shaft fractures with soft tissue injury

average of 28.2 weeks was required. These figures serve to reemphasize the importance of biomechanical factors in the successful operative management of fractures using a plate.

From a biomechanical and biological standpoint, plate fixation offers important advantages in the treatment of tibial shaft fractures with soft tissue injury (Schweiberer et al. 1975). Through accurate reduction and the establishment of interfragmental compression, it is possible to obtain intimate contact between the bone ends and maintain this contact in a highly stable configuration. This hastens the revascularization of devitalized cortical bone and denuded fragments while allowing fracture union to proceed undisturbed (Olerud, Dankwarth-Lilieström 1971; Rhinelander 1974; Schweiberer et al. 1974).

The vascular damage caused by the presence of the plate and the fixation screws is minimal. Consequently, the adverse biological effects of the fixation material are slight (Rhinelander 1980).

Plate fixation should be utilized only if the following conditions apply:

1. **It must be possible to attach the plate under cover of viable soft tissue.**
2. **Application of the plate must entail minimal soft tissue dissection.**
3. **The implant must be applied in a biomechanically optimal fashion so that a stable fixation is obtained.**

1) Plate Position. Plates that are exposed or covered by soft tissue of doubtful viability are very often a nidus for infection. Thus, a viable soft tissue coverage is an important prerequisite for compression plating. The standard site for tibial plating is the lateral surface of the bone, because skin lesions of the lower leg occur most frequently on the anteromedial side (Fig. 8). The muscles of the anterior compartment are carefully released from their loose attachments with the bone. The periosteum should be left in place, for it derives its main blood supply from the anterior tibial artery and contributes to cortical nutrition.

Lateral plating is favorable not only in terms of muscle coverage but also from a biomechanical standpoint, in that the posteriorally-directed bending forces tend to act in the plane of the highest plate stiffness (Fig. 9a).

Posterior plating of the tibia has a very limited application, for it entails considerable soft tissue trauma and denudation of the bone. It should be considered only in cases where a posteromedial approach is dictated by soft tissue damage confined essentially to the posterior aspect of the lower leg, and little additional stripping of soft tissue from the bone is required (see Fig. 12 in Tscherne). This placement is also unfavorable biomechanically, because the implant is subjected to large bending stresses, creating a high risk of complications such as instability (Fig. 9b) and plate damage. In 160 of our own cases, the plate was applied laterally in 122 cases, medially in 21, and posteriorly in 17. Based on our negative experience with posterior plating as well as that of our authors (Rüter et al. 1978), we have concluded that posterior plating has very limited indications, indeed, and should be done under the conditions outlined above.

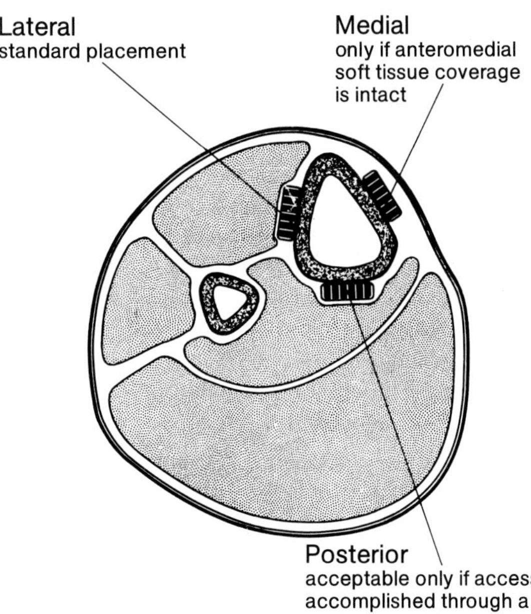

Fig. 8. Sites of plate application for tibial shaft fractures with soft tissue injury

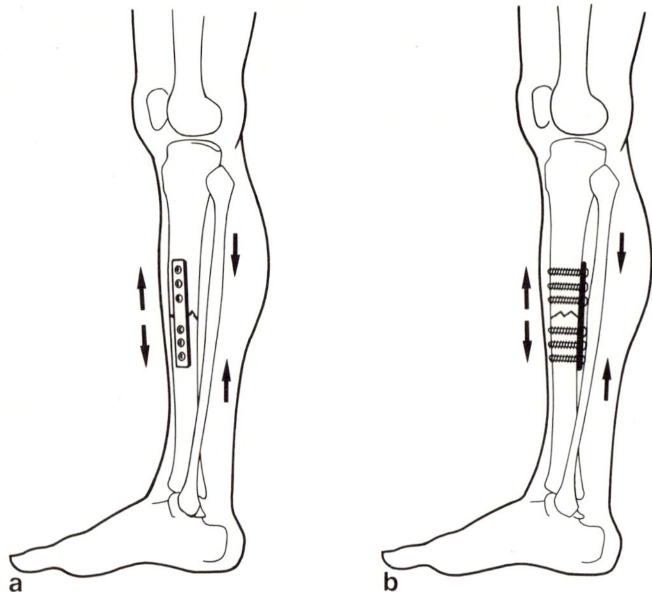

Fig. 9a, b. Biomechanically favorable lateral (**a**) and unfavorable posterior (**b**) plating of the tibial shaft

2) Bone Viability. Any stripping of soft tissues that goes beyond that already caused by the trauma will impair the vascularity and healing ability of the bone. It will also predispose the bone to infection. This is particularly true of fragments with primarily intact soft tissue investment. Thus, the indications for plate fixation frequently are limited by biological considerations. Plating should not be done if it would require exposing the only bony surface that still has its soft tissue attachments, and long sections of circumferential denudation would result.

With comminuted fractures, stabilizing the fracture site by means of a bridging technique may be the best way of preserving fragment viability. This cannot be achieved by plating alone.

On the other hand, if the bone has already been denuded of soft tissue by the trauma, and applying the plate would require no significant additional exposure, a stable internal fixation based on interfragmental compression will create the most favorable conditions for fragment revitalization and fracture consolidation.

3) Biomechanics and Fixation Technique. Compression plating is a highly demanding procedure which requires a high level of biomechanical knowledge and technical proficiency. Bone healing is extremely susceptible to disruptive mechanical influences, and even a micro-instability can seriously interfere with ossifying processes (Willenegger, Perren, Schenk 1971).

Given the special situation of the tibia, which shows marked local variations of strength and of geometry, the absence of a constant tension side, and a tendency toward severe fracture configurations, the implants must be applied in a biomechanically optimal fashion if a stable fixation of the fragments is to be obtained.

The narrow AO dynamic compression plate (DCP) has proved especially useful (Allgöwer, Perren 1980). This implant has several important advantages: Axial compression can be effected with the screws alone or by means of a separate tension device, there is no problem of uncontrolled compression losses during insertion of the screws, and the plate perforations allow a variable screw placement (Allgöwer et al. 1973).

In terms of mechanical properties, the plate is characterized by a low bending resistance and a low fatique strength under repeated bending loads. Failure of the plate invariably occurs at one of its perforations. For a realistic assessment of the mechanical capabilities of the narrow DCP, it must be considered that each perforation reduces the cross-sectional area of the plate by 42%, and that the resistance moment (the main determinant of bending strength) at a perforation is only 37% of that in the middle plate segment (Gotzen 1978) (Fig. 10). From this it is clear that the plate is incapable of functioning as a solitary load-bearing member, and that stability can be achieved only in conjunction with a buttressing bony element or by means of supplementary fixation.

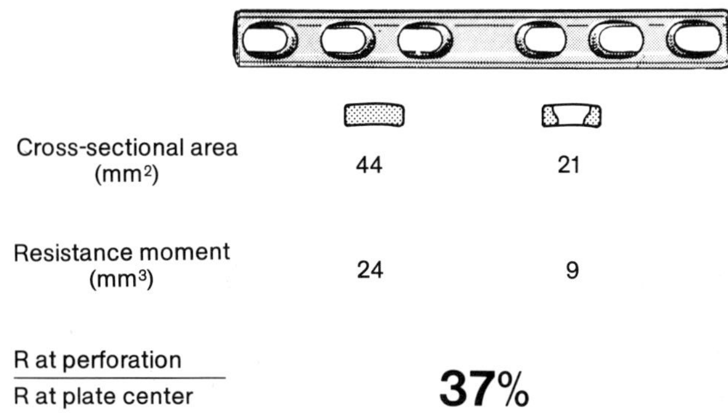

Fig. 10. Cross-sectional geometry of the narrow DCP at a perforation and between perforations, with the corresponding resistance moments

Fragment fixation utilizing interfragmental compression is the most effective form of stabilization (Danis 1949; Müller, Allgöwer, Schneider, Willenegger 1977). In torsion fractures and long oblique fractures, internal fixation with lag screws and a neutralization plate is a simple but effective technique. Instability frequently develops in more transversely-oriented fractures (Karlström, Olerud 1974; Thunold et al. 1976) and in cases where residual transverse or oblique fracture surfaces are left following lag screw fixation of isolated fragments.

The stabilizing effect of interfragmentary compression against bending loads is based on the preloading of the fracture surfaces, while stabilization against torsional loads is based upon the static friction that exists between the fracture surfaces (Perren, Hayes 1974). This stability is present only when compression is applied across the entire fracture site.

Axial compression of this type cannot be obtained simply by applying tension to the plate when attaching it to the bone (Aeberhard 1973; Perren, Hays 1974; Claudi 1979; Gotzen et al. 1980). The torque resulting from the eccentric application of force is compensated by overbending of the plate, which leads to an asymmetric longitudinal compression of the bone, with compressive stresses concentrated in a small area directly beneath the plate. Always small loads cause interfragmentary motion in an osteosynthesis with such a biomechanical constellation. To produce nearly uniform compressive contact stresses across the fracture site, and thus achieve an effective interfragmental preload and friction, it is necessary to prebend the plate before it is applied (Bagby 1958; Perren, Hayes 1974; Müller et al. 1977; Gotzen et al. 1981).

The importance of prebending in clinical practice is demonstrated by an analysis of our own cases. In the 34 plate fixations that were biomechanically flawed, a lack of prebending was the principal or contributing cause of instability-related complications in 24 cases.

The process of applying tension to a prebent plate can be divided into three phases (Gotzen et al. 1980, 1981) (Fig. 11). In phase I, the point of interfragmental contact and the focal point of compression are located in the cortex opposite the plate. The bend-back moment of the plate increases in proportion to the amount of tension applied. When the

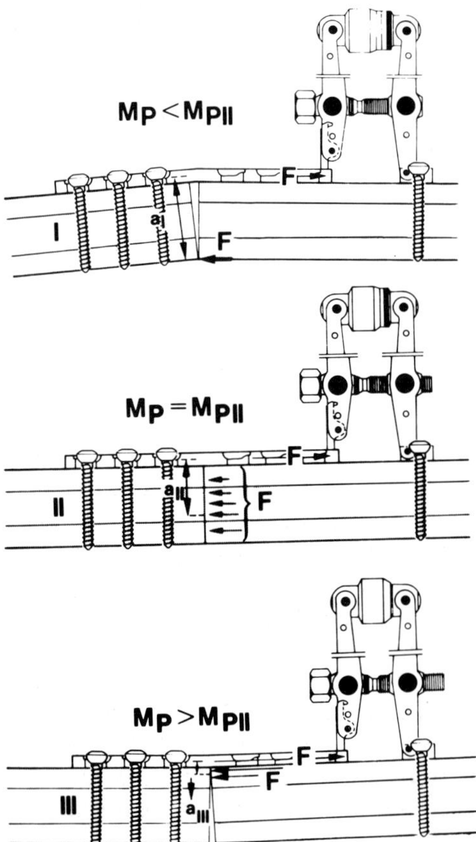

Fig. 11. The three phases of applying tension to a prebent plate

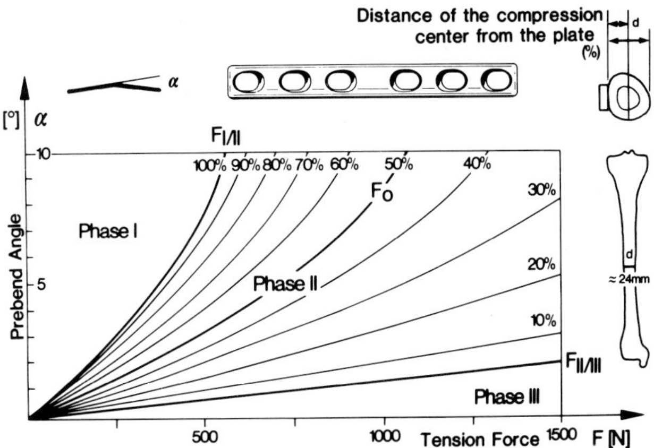

Fig. 12. Graphic representation of the phases of compression obtained with the prebent narrow DCP on the tibia shaft

primary bend in the plate has been effaced and interfragmental contact is complete, phase II begins. The main point of the compression shifts toward the plate, and the bend-back moment of the plate remains constant. If tension on the plate is further increased to levels not ordinarily achieved in practice, a third phase is reached in which the fragments gape in the side opposite the plate.

The contact pressure between the fragments, and thus the primary preload and static friction for stability, are dependent upon the bend-back moment of the plate in phase II. The greater the prebend angle of the plate, the greater the bend-back moment. The amount of tension applied to the plate after phase II is reached has little additional influence on stability. The diagram in Fig. 12 illustrates the correlations between prebending and primary tension as well as the distribution of compression.

Prebend angles of 4° to 8°, depending on the mechanical quality of the buttressing bone, are recommended for an effective stabilization. When the prebending technique is used, it is better to apply tension to the plate with the aid of a separate device than to rely on the plate's self-compressing capability. The tension device with a built-in force meter enables tension to be applied in a precise, quantitative fashion. In addition, this device has a travel sufficient to ensure that phase II is safely reached. The tension device also allows greater flexibility and room for correction when the fixation is performed.

Another useful stabilizing technique is to insert a lag screw obliquely through the plate such that it crosses the fracture line (Müller et al. 1977; Claudi 1979; Gotzen et al. 1981). The contribution of the oblique lag screw to stability depends largely on how it is placed. It must pass approximately through the center of the interfragmental plane, and it must securely engage the opposite cortex. This must be considered at the time the plate is applied. Excellent stability can be achieved by combining the prebending technique with an oblique lag screw. The interfragmental contact pressure produced by the primary bend increases in proportion to the perpendicular force exerted by the lag screw on the fracture surfaces (Fig. 13).

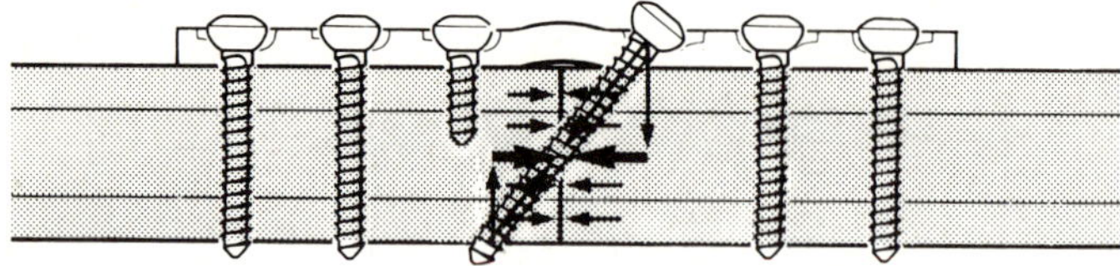

Fig. 13. Mechanical result of combining a prebent plate with a lag screw inserted through the plate

The results of biomechanical studies in this area are presented in Fig. 14. The influence of prebending and oblique lag screw insertion on bending stability is clearly demonstrated. Clinical applications are illustrated in Figs. 15 and 16.

Special problems arise if, following the reduction, the bony buttress is found to be deficient, or the fracture surfaces are not compressible as a result of comminution. If the defect is located beneath the plate and the opposite cortex provides an adequate buttress, stability can still be achieved by utilizing the prebending technique (Fig. 17).

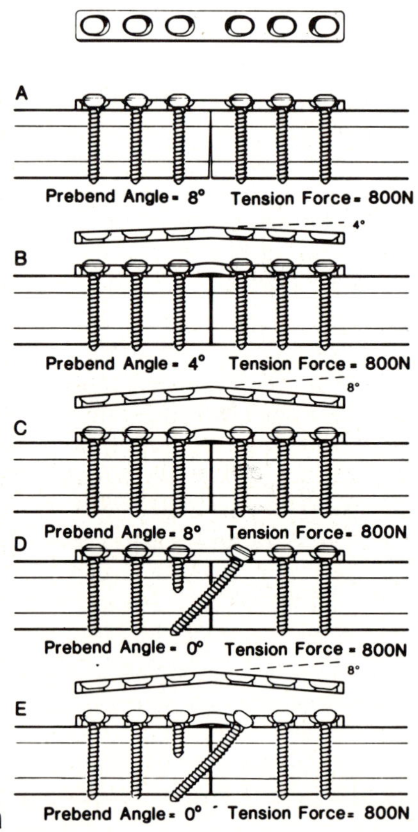

Fig. 14a, b. Examples showing various ways of applying a narrow DCP to a transverse tibial shaft osteotomy (a) and the corresponding load diagram demonstrating the importance of a prebent plate and oblique lag screw for stability (b)

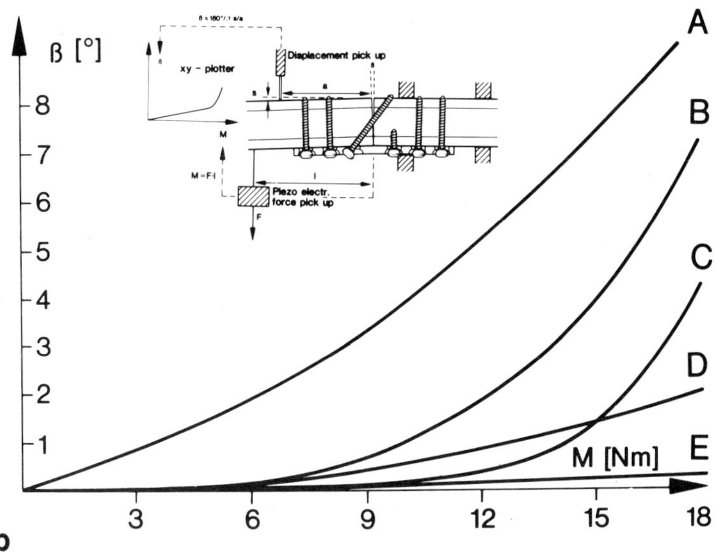

Fig. 14b

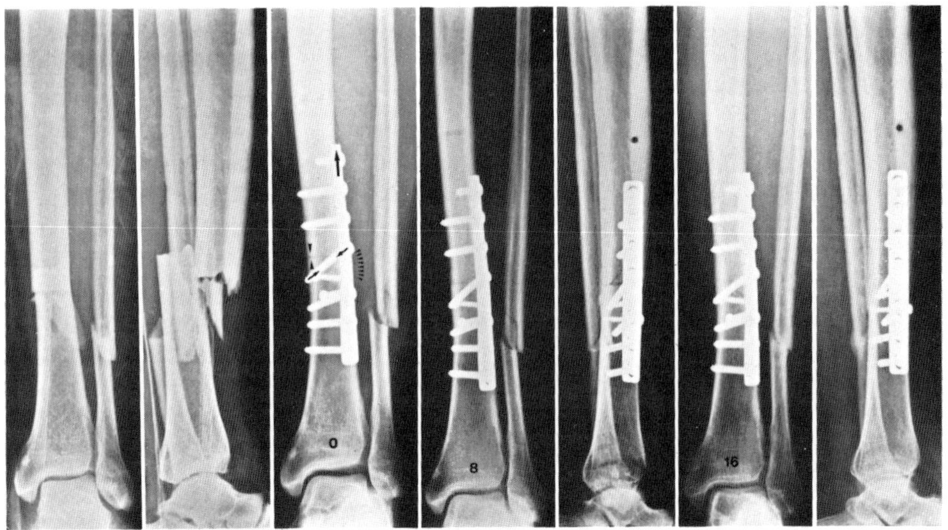

Fig. 15. Plate fixation of a grade III open tibial shaft fracture incorporating a large devitalized fragment. Optimum stability and complication-free healing are ensured by prebending the plate, using the tension device, and inserting an oblique lag screw through the plate

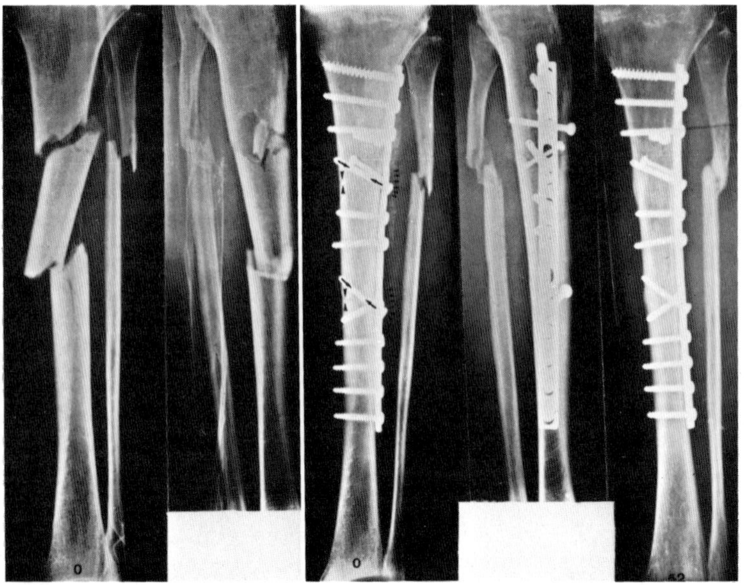

Fig. 16. Plate fixation of a grade II open segmental tibial shaft fracture. Stability and healing are promoted by prebending the plate over both fractures and using oblique lag screws

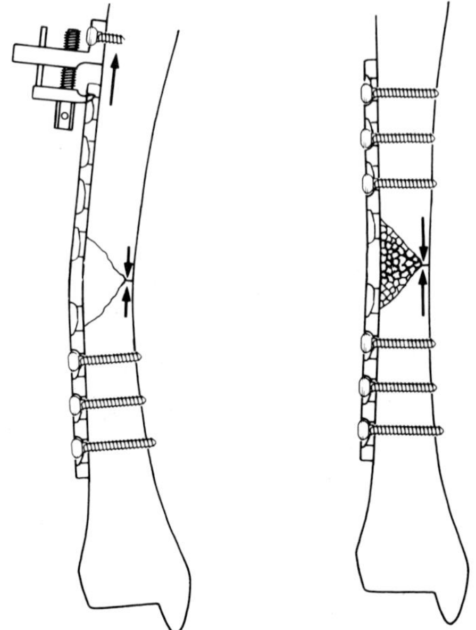

Fig. 17. Use of the prebending technique to achieve stability with an intact bony buttress on the side opposite the plate

In cases where the bone ends are in contact only beneath the plate, or a significant defect is created by a loss of bone substance, the plate must function as a solitary load-bearing member and will not provide the necessary stability. In these cases, supplementary fixation is indicated.

If soft-tissue condition permit a plate to be applied medially, then supplementary plating of the fibula is often an effective means of enhancing the stability of mid- and distal-third tibial fractures, relieving stress on the primary plate (Gotzen et al. 1978), and providing the mechanical rest at the fracture site necessary for osseous healing (Fig. 18a, Fig. 19).

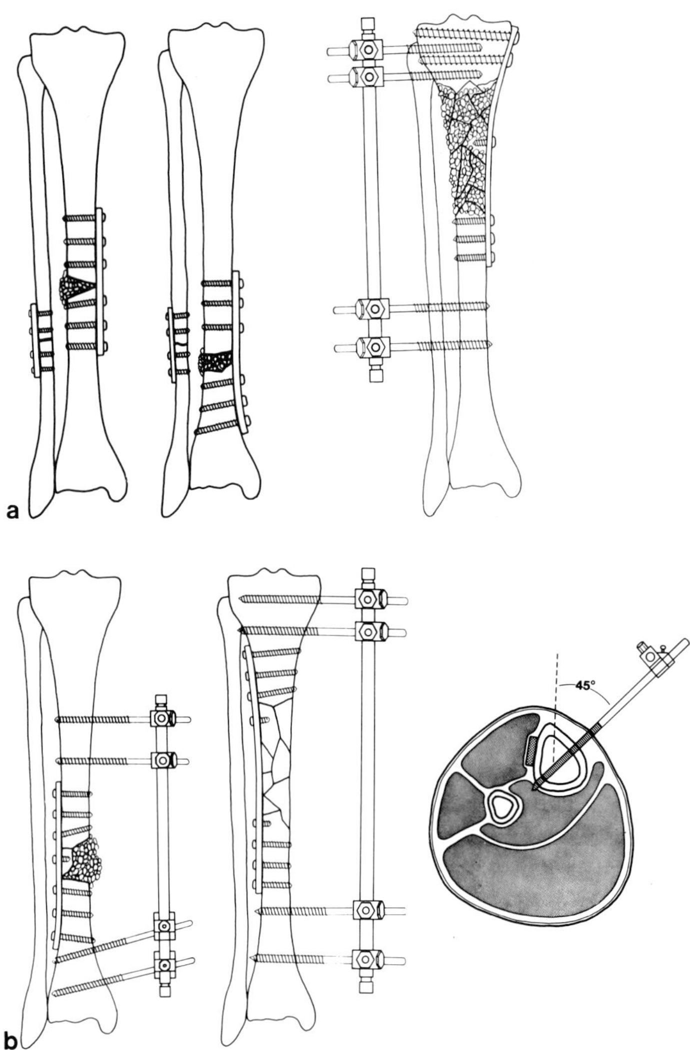

Fig. 18a, b. Plate fixation of tibial shaft fractures for which supplementary stabilization is recommended. **a** A medial plate is supplemented by plating the fibula (distal and mid-third fractures) or by applying an external half frame anterolaterally (proximal fractures). **b** A lateral plate is supplemented by an anteromedial half frame

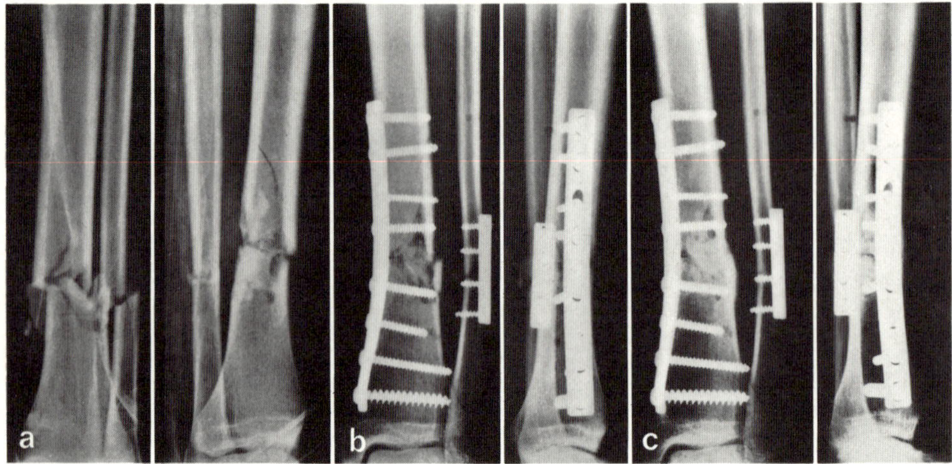

Fig. 19. **a** Grade I open comminuted fracture of the distal tibial shaft. **b** The plate on the medial tibia had to be supplemented with a fibular plate due to lack of a bony buttress. Primary grafting was done with autologous cancellous bone. **c** Full weight bearing was possible at 16 weeks

A lateral plate or a medial plate on a high tibial fracture is effectively supplemented by applying an external half-frame to the side opposite the plate. The frame should be offset 45° from the frontal plate. The external fixation is removed when fracture union has progressed well enough that instability and plate fracture are no longer a danger. This procedure is also recommended for lengthy comminuted fractures if soft tissue conditions permit. To preserve fragment viability, the fixation should be applied in a "bridging" configuration. The plate is screwed to the main fragments such that a correct bone length and axial alignment are obtained. Individual fragments in the comminuted zone may be fixed to the plate with lag screws (Fig. 18b).

External Fixation

The external fixator has become an indispensable tool for solving the many problems related to tibial shaft fractures with severe soft tissue injuries. Biomechanical improvements in frame designs have made external stabilization a highly reliable fixation technique.

The main advantages of external fixation are its relative technical simplicity and its minimal biological interference with injured tissues. The implants may be inserted away from the fracture site, and exposure can be kept to the minimum necessary for debridement of the soft tissues and bone.

The main disadvantages of external fixation in a biological sense are the frequent lack of interfragmental contact and the inability of an external frame to effect an absolutely stable fixation. These deficiencies lead to disturbances of revascularization and account for the delayed fracture union that is frequently observed.

External fixation is mainly indicated for fractures that are not amenable to plate fixation.

We believe that external stabilization is urgently indicated in the following situations:

1. **When soft tissue injuries are very severe, and the prime concern is salvage of the extremity.**
2. **When a plate cannot be covered with viable soft tissue.**
3. **When plating would necessitate extensive devascularization of the bone.**
4. **When plating cannot provide effective stabilization.**

In major lower leg trauma it is common for several of these situations to coexist. However, only one needs to be present in order to contraindicate plate fixation.

Situation 1: In many fractures with grade III open or closed soft tissue injuries, the main concern is to save the extremity. Operative stabilization of the fracture is done mainly to encourage soft tissue healing and avoid infection (Kull, Rittmann 1981). Gunshot fracture and fractures with a high level of primary contamination are included in this category. Fracture union is usually a secondary priority, and in most cases definitive fracture care is deferred until a later date. In these extreme situations, external fixation is the treatment of choice owing to its minimal adverse biological effects, its biomechanical reliability, and the rapidity and ease with which it can be applied.

Situations 2 and 3: The grounds for use of the external fixator in the section on Plate Fixation.

Situation 4: If soft tissue conditions do not prohibit plate fixation, but the fracture configuration is such that it cannot be stably immobilized by that method, plating should not be performed.

Thus, plating is contraindicated for fractures with significant bone loss, complex segmental fractures, and for most extensive comminuted fractures. These include periarticular comminuted fractures, in which stable fixation of the fragments is frequently impossible. External fixation, applied across the joint if necessary, gives better stability and entails substantially less surgical trauma. Plating is also contraindicated when bone strength is seriously impaired by osteoporosis or other disease, because the screws do not hold well in weak bone. Also, quite apart from conditions at the site of injury, there may be extentuating circumstances which would favor external fixation over internal fixation because of the fewer risks involved.

For the surgeon who has had little experience with plate fixation, external fixation offers a valuable alternative. If complications arise, they are usually easier to control than those associated with internal plating. In unreliable patients such as alcoholics and drug addicts, as well as in multiply injured patients with head trauma whose operated limb may be subject to considerable stresses during postoperative care, the advantages of the external fixator are equally apparent. Time constraints in the face of multiple injuries may also favor external fixation in the polytrauma victim.

After the external fixator has been applied, there is still the option of changing to other treatment modalities once the soft tissues are under control, or if such a change is warranted on social or pathophysiologic grounds.

Biomechanics and Fixation Technique

The "tent frame" configuration designed by Hierholzer in 1975 and consisting of Steinmann pins (transfixing pins) and Schanz screws (threaded half pins) has found wide acceptance as an external fixation technique. Regardless of whether interfragmental compression or limb length retention is the goal, the correct placement and primary stressing (bowing) of the implants have an important influence on the stability that is achieved (Hierholzer et al. 1978; Martinek et al. 1980; Müller, Witzel 1981; Kleining 1981). The two Steinmann pins in each fragment should be spaced well apart from each other, and the Schanz screws should be inserted close to the fracture site.

The manner in which the transfixing pins are bowed is determined by the quality of the bony buttress. If the interfragmental contact zone is judged to be pressure-competent, then the fracture may be stabilized under axial compression. In this case each set of Steinmann pins is bowed toward the fracture, so that the spring tension of the pins exerts a compressive force across the fracture line. If limb length retention is the main objective,

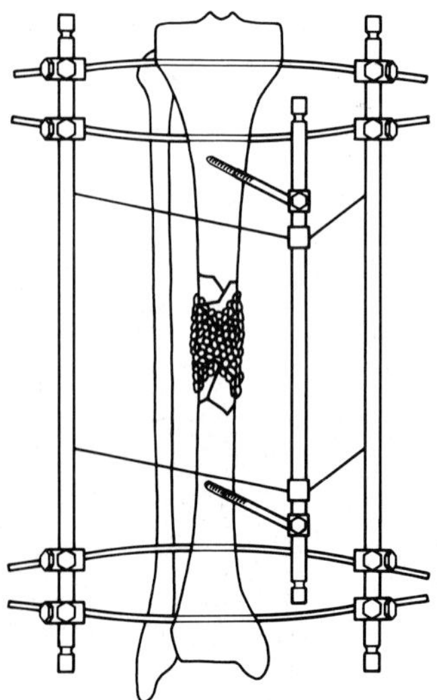

Fig. 20. External fixator assembled in a tent configuration to maintain a normal bone length until union can occur. The Steinmann pins in the main fragments are bowed for added stability and are supplemented by half pins (Schanz screws) inserted close to the fracture

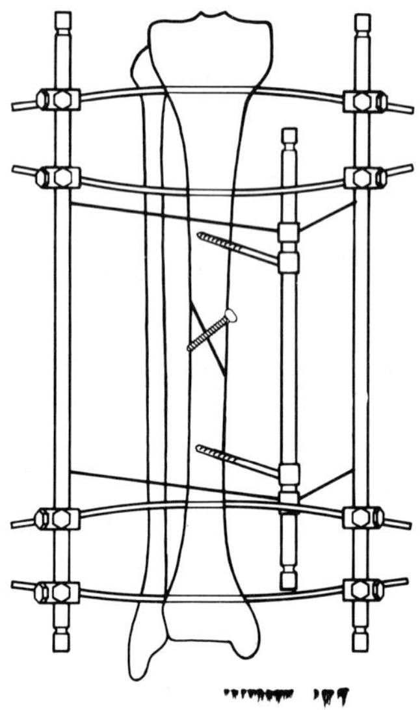

Fig. 21. Stabilization with an external fixator and lag screw – a favorable combination for oblique fracture surfaces

rather than axial compression, the pins in the same fragment are bowed toward each other (Figs. 20 and 22). Besides enhancing stability, bowing of the transfixing pins is an effective way to prevent the implants from loosening in the bone. In fractures with oblique surfaces, stability and healing conditions can be significantly enhanced by combining the external fixation with interfragmental screw fixation (Claes et al. 1979) (Figs. 21 and 23).

The main disadvantages of frames mounted in the frontal plane are the significant soft tissue trauma, especially from muscle impalement (vascular injury, painful and perhaps permanent functional deficit, infection), and the large distance between the bone and connecting rods, which lessens stability. As a solution, Burri and Claes (1981) recommend an anteromedial V-shaped frame with a total of 4 Schanz screws in each main fragment (2 anterior and 2 medial) and 4 cross-bars mounted between the main connecting rods. In their biomechanical studies, these authors were able to achieve a stability that matched that of the tent configuration.

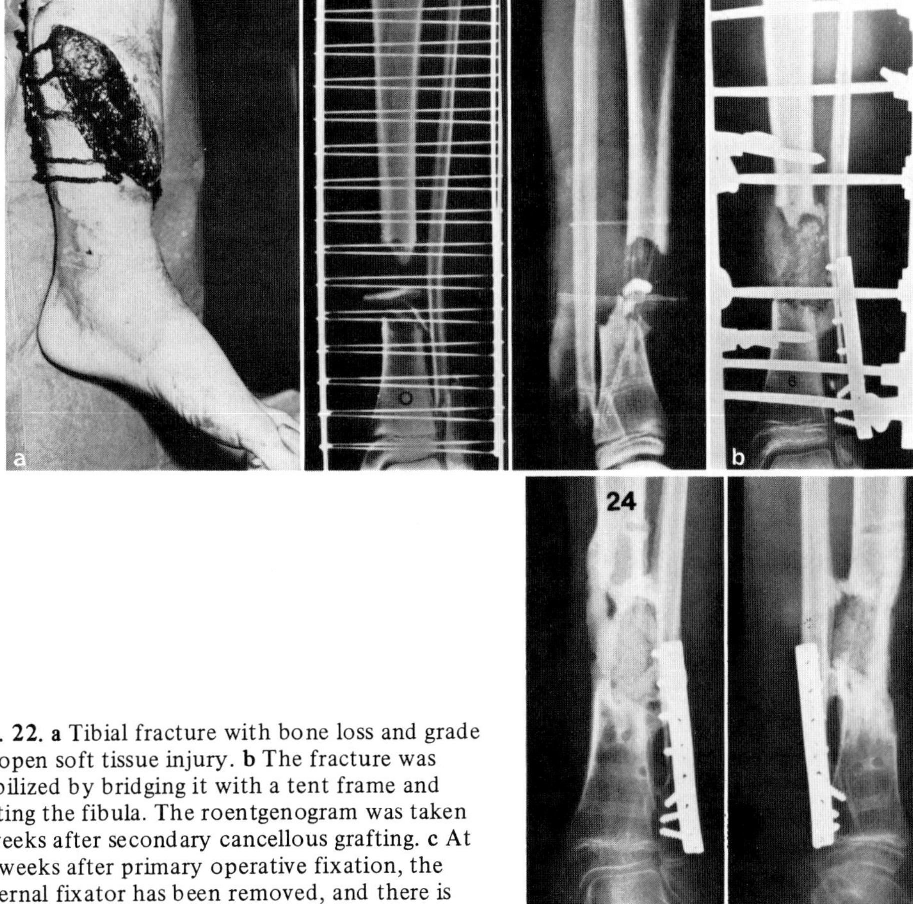

Fig. 22. a Tibial fracture with bone loss and grade III open soft tissue injury. **b** The fracture was stabilized by bridging it with a tent frame and plating the fibula. The roentgenogram was taken 6 weeks after secondary cancellous grafting. **c** At 24 weeks after primary operative fixation, the external fixator has been removed, and there is bony consolidation of the fracture

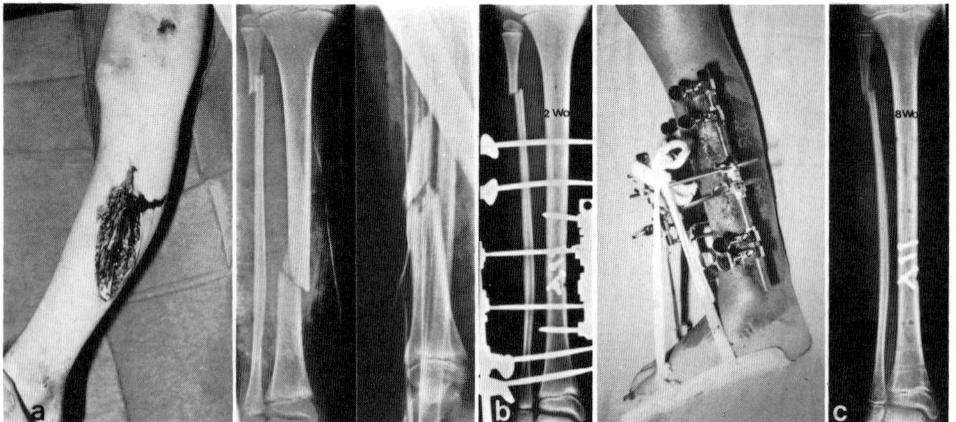

Fig. 23. **a** Grade II open segmental tibial shaft fracture stabilized by interfragmental screw fixation and a tent frame. **b** Shows the situation at 2 weeks. **c** At 8 weeks the external fixation was removed

In an effort to further reduce soft tissue trauma and shorten the distance between the bone and connecting rods, while also reducing the number of implants and simplifying asssembly, we have developed a unilateral half frame for anterior application. The device is assembled by inserting two Schanz screws into each main fragment from the anterior side and interconnecting them by means of an rectangular rod equipped with special fixation clamps.

Discoveries made in experimental stability studies (Schlenzka, Gotzen, Warmbold 1982; Warmbold, Gotzen, Schlenzka 1982) may be summarized as follows as they relate to the application of the anterior half frame:

1. The distance between rod and bone should be minimal. Owing to the sparse anterior soft tissue coverage of the tibia, this distance can be reduced to 3–4 cm.
2. The two central Schanz screws should be inserted as close to the fracture as possible.
3. A maximum distance should be maintained between the Schanz screws in each main fragment, though no additional stability is gained beyond 6 cm.

Primary stress in the system is created in much the same way as in a full-frame configuration. If a bony buttress is present, the two central Schanz screws are bowed toward each other to exert interfragmental compression. The two peripheral screws are bowed slightly inward or outward to lock them in place. In a bridging (length-retaining) configuration, the screws in each main fragment are bowed in opposite directions, either toward or away from each other. A further advantage of the system is that it enables a dynamic external splinting with neutralization of bending and rotation movements through removal of the locking screws in the fixation clamps on one fracture side (Fig. 24). Clinical use of the anterior half frame is illustrated in Fig. 25.

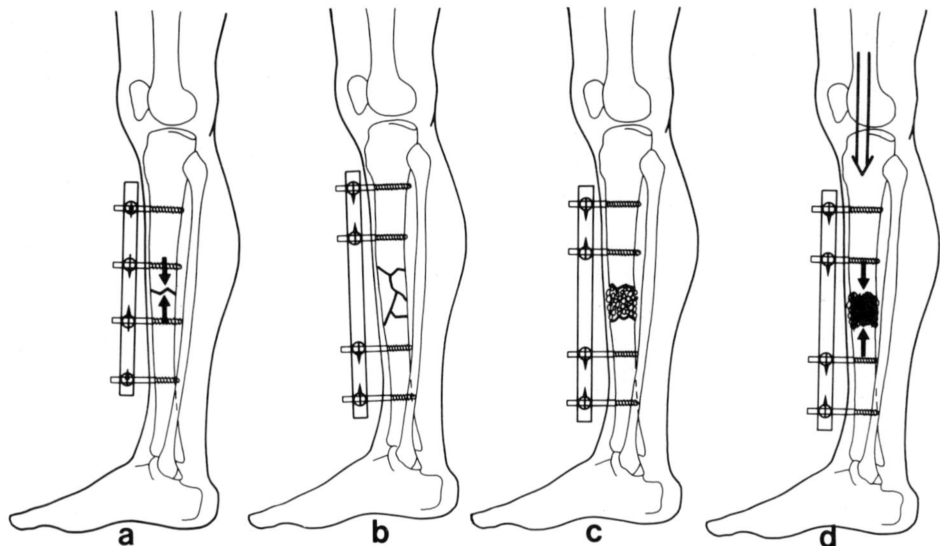

Fig. 24a–d. Half frame (Monofixateur) placed to the anterior surface of the tibia. Excellent stability is achieved by the proximity of the pin clamps to the bone, the biomechanically correct placement of the Schanz screws and bowing of the screws. **a** Configuration for exerting axial compression. **b** Configuration for fracture neutralization. **c** Configuration for bone length retention. **d** Configuration for dynamization

Conclusions

The lower leg is by far the most common site of combined injuries to bone and soft tissue. Functional recovery of the often severely traumatized extremity requires optimum therapy. To maximize the chances of uneventful soft tissue and fracture healing, the following principles of treatment should be rigorously observed.

1. **Meticulous wound debridement.**
2. **Atraumatic operating technique that preserves tissue viability.**
3. **Primary, stable operative fixation of the fracture.**
4. **Decompression of the soft tissues.**
5. **Soft tissue coverage of exposed bone.**

1) Wound Debridement: This includes the meticulous cleansing of the wound and the removal of all irreversibly damaged soft tissues and useless devitalized bone fragments.

2) Atraumatic Operating Technique. Exposure and treatment of the fracture must be done as atraumatically as possible to avoid exacerbating the primary damage and thus further jeopardizing the vascularity and viability of the bone and soft tissues.

3) Primary Stable Operative Fixation. Operative stabilization is done by the method most appropriate for the given situation in order to meet the requirement of stable fragment

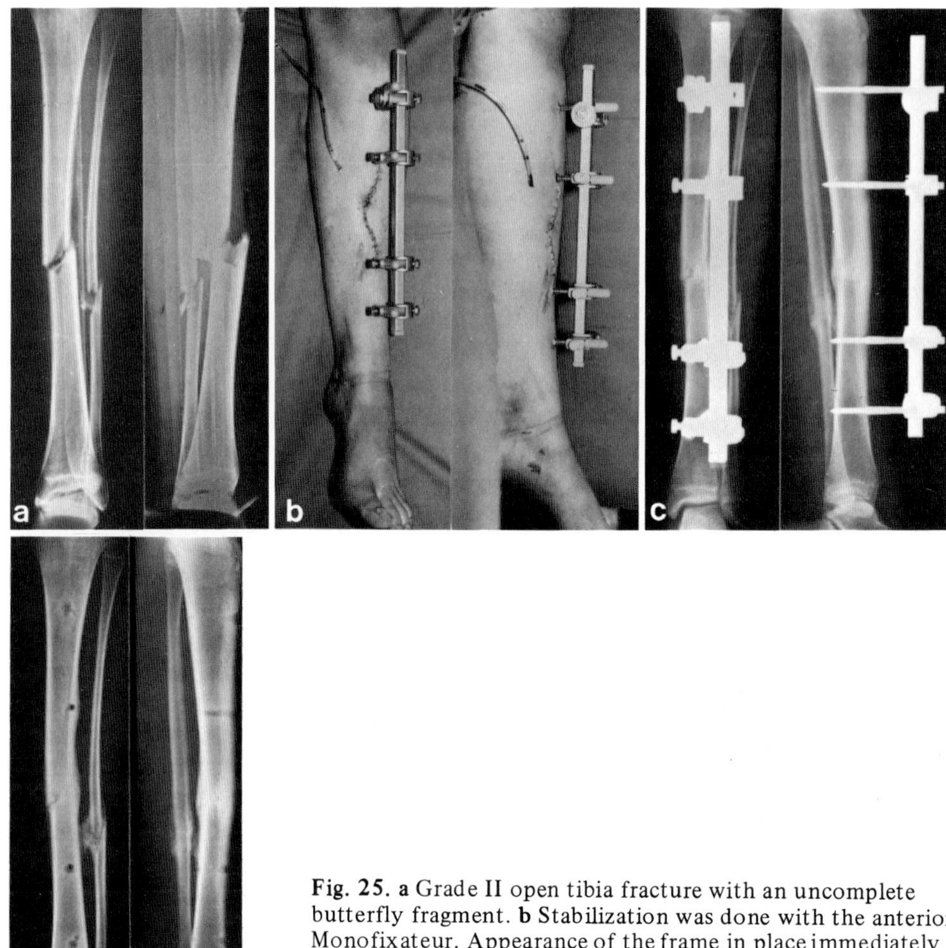

Fig. 25. a Grade II open tibia fracture with an uncomplete butterfly fragment. b Stabilization was done with the anterior Monofixateur. Appearance of the frame in place immediately after surgery. c Bone healing progressed rapidly with visible callus formation through dynamization of the fixator one week after application. d At 10 weeks the fracture was consolidated and the fixator was removed

fixation without critically endangering bone and soft tissue viability. Thus, the selection of the fixation method and the fixation technique must be based upon a thorough assessment of the nature and localization of soft tissue and osseous lesions, and of the biomechanical aspects and potential adverse biological effects of the various stabilization methods.

Intramedullary Nailing

This procedure should be limited to "nailable" fractures associated with grade I soft tissue injury, and to fractures with grade II soft tissue injury in which there is no significant denudation of the fragments. Reaming of the medullary canal should be avoided if at all possible or at least kept to a moderate level so that intramedullary trauma can be minimized. During closed nailing, fracture hematoma and reaming debris are flushed out through a separate incision.

Plate Fixation

Plate fixation is suitable when the plate can be attached under cover of viable tissue, application of the plate does not entail extensive denudation of the bone, and a stable fixation can be obtained. Plating is most commonly utilized for fractures with moderate soft tissue injuries. The lateral tibial surface is the standard site of application. To obtain interfragmental compression, the plates must be adequately prebent and applied under tension. An oblique lag screw should also be inserted through the plate whenever possible. If compressible surfaces are lacking due to absence of a bony buttress, stability can nevertheless be obtained by applying an external half frame opposite the plate or, for mid- and distal-third fractures that are medially plated, by supplementary plating of the fibula.

External Fixation

External fixation is mandatory in the presence of severe soft tissue and bony lesions (grade III soft tissue damage associated with segmental fractures, commitued fractures, or fractures with bone loss; gunshot fractures, heavy primary contamination) when infection prophylaxis and soft tissue healing are of primary concern in order to save the extremity. Fracture union in such cases is usually a deferable goal. Even with milder soft tissue trauma and simpler fracture configurations, external fixation provides a low-risk alternative to compression plating in unreliable patients and for surgeons who are unfamiliar with the plating technique. For the tubular external fixation system of the ASIF, the tent configuration is standard. In oblique fractures, stability and bone healing can be significantly improved by supplementary screw fixation of the fragments.

The anterior half frame (Monofixateur) with its two Schanz screws inserted into each main fragment offers an excellent means of reducing soft tissue trauma and simplifying assembly. The small distance between the bone and rod and optimum placement of the screws create a highly stable configuration. Dynamization promotes fracture healing.

4) Decompression of Soft Tissues. In the face of pronounced tissue swelling, the best way to improve tissue perfusion is to incise the fascia, leave the skin open and, if necessary, apply relaxing incisions. Neglect of these measures is an invitation to posttraumatic ischemic syndrome with its severe acute effects (necrosis of muscle and skin, infection) and late changes (loss of function, contractures).

5) Soft Tissue Coverage of Exposed Bone. Small areas of exposed surface of the tibia, can be covered primarily with adjacent muscle. If the exposure is extensive, early secondary plastic measures should be undertaken following transitory coverage with synthetic skin.

References

1. Aeberhard J (1973) Einfluß der Plattenüberbiegung auf die Torsionsstabilität der Osteosynthese. Dissertation, Bern
2. Allgöwer M (1971) Weichteilprobleme und Infektionsrisiko der Osteosynthese. Langenbecks Arch Chir 329:1127
3. Allgöwer M, Kinzl L, Matter P, Perren SM, Rüedi T (1973) The Dynamic Compression Plate (DCP). Springer, Berlin Heidelberg New York
4. Allgöwer M, Perren SM (1980) Operating of tibial shaft fractures. Unfallheilkd 83: 214
5. Brooker AF, Edwards CH (1979) External Fixation. Williams & Wilkins, Baltimore
6. Brookes M (1971) The blood supply to bone. Butterworth, London
7. Burri C, Claes L (1981) Indikation und Formen der Anwendung des Fixateur externe am Unterschenkel. Unfallheilkd 84:177
8. Claes L, Burri C, Heckmann G, Rüter A (1979) Biomechanische Untersuchungen zur Stabilität von Tibiaosteosynthesen mit dem Fixateur externe und einer Minimalosteosynthese. Akt Traumatol 9:185
9. Claudi BF (1979) Untersuchungen zur Frage der Stabilitätsverbesserung von Druckplattenosteosynthesen durch schräge Plattenzugschraube und Plattenüberbiegung. Habilitation, München
10. Crock HV (1967) The blood supply of the lower limb bones in man. Livingstone, London Edinburgh
11. Danis R (1949) Theorie et practique de l'osteosynthese. Masson, Paris
12. Eitel F (1981) Indikation zur operativen Frakturbehandlung. Hefte Unfallheilkd 154
13. Göthmann L (1961) Arterial changes in experimental fractures of the monkeys tibia treated with intramedullary nailing. Acta Chir Scand 121:56
14. Gotzen L (1978) Die Plattenosteosynthese am Knochenschaft – Rückblick auf die Entwicklung und aktuelle Forschung. Tagungsbericht 19. Unfallseminar, Hannover
15. Gotzen L, Haas N, Hütter J, Köller W (1978) Die Bedeutung der Fibula für die Stabilität der Plattenosteosynthese an der Tibia. Unfallheilkd 81:409
16. Gotzen L, Hütter J, Haas N (1980) Die Kompressionsosteosynthese am Knochenschaft – Biomechanische Untersuchungen zur Plattenvorbiegung und Vorspannung. Unfallchirurgie 6:14
17. Gotzen L, Haas N, Strohfeld G (1981) Zur Biomechanik der Plattenosteosynthese. Schräge Plattenzugschraube-Plattenvorbierung. Unfallheilkd 84:439
18. Gotzen L, Haas N, Strohfeld G (1981) Experimentelle und praktische Grundlagen zur Vorbiegung der schmalen und breiten AO-Platte (DCP). Unfallheilkd 84:121
19. Hierholzer G (1975) Stabilisierung des Knochenbruches mit Weichteilschaden mit Fixateur externe. Langenbecks Arch Chir 339:505
20. Hierholzer G, Kleining R, Hörster G, Zemedies P (1978) External fixation. Arch Orthop Traumat Surg 92:175
21. Hildebrandt G (1979) Die Bedeutung der periossären und intramedullären Durchblutung für die Entstehung der posttraumatischen Osteomyelitis und für die Wahl des Osteosyntheseverfahrens. Beitr Orthop Traumatol 26:181
22. Holden CEA (1974) Traumatic tension ischaemia in muscles. Injury 5:223
23. Holden CEA (1979) The pathology and prevention of Volkmann's contracture. J Bone Joint Surg 61B:296
24. Karlström G, Olerud S (1977) Stable external fixation of open tibial fractures. Orthopaedic Review 8:25
25. Karlström G, Olerud S (1974) Fractures of the tibial shaft. Clin Orthop 105:82
26. Kimura T (1974) Mechanical characteristics of human lower leg bones. J Faculty Science, Univ of Tokyo, Vol 4
27. Klasen HJ, Binnendyk B (1982) Soft-tissue injury and fasciotomy. Injury 14:58
28. Knapp U, Weller S (1978) Weichteilversorgung bei offenen Frakturen. Akt Traumatol 8:319

29. Küntscher G (1962) Praxis der Marknagelung. Schattauer, Stuttgart
30. Kull CH, Rittmann WW (1981) Der Fixateur externe als Stabilisierungsverfahren in Extremsituationen frischer oder kompliziert verlaufender Frakturen. Helv Chir Acta 48:661
31. v Lanz P, Wachsmuth W (1972) Praktische Anatomie I/IV, Bein und Statik. Springer, Berlin Heidelberg New York
32. Lawyer R (1979) Treatment of complex tibial fractures. In: Brooker AF, Edwards CHC (eds) External Fixation. Williams & Wilkins, Baltimore
33. Macnab J, de Haas WG (1974) The role of periostal blood supply in the healing of fractures of the tibia. Clin Orthop 105:27
34. Martinek H, Egkher E, Wielke B (1980) Experimentelle Grundlagen zur optimalen Montageform äußerer Spanner. Hefte Unfallheilkd 148:516
35. Müller KH, Witzel U (1981) Die Fixateur externe Osteosynthese ohne knöcherne Abstützung an der unteren Gliedmaße. Arch Orthop Traumat Surg 99:117
36. Müller ME, Allgöwer M, Schneider R, Willenegger H (1977) Manual der Osteosynthese. 2. Aufl. Springer, Berlin Heidelberg New York
37. Nelson G, Kelly PJ, Petersen LFA, Janes JM (1960). Blood supply of the human tibia. J Bone Surg 42A:645
38. Olerud S, Danckwardt-Lilleström G (1971) Fracture healing in compression osteosynthesis. Acta Orthop Scand (Suppl) 137
39. Perren SM, Hayes WC (1974) Biomechanik der Plattenosteosynthese. Med Orthop Tech 2:56
40. Rehn J, Katthagen BD (1980) Osteosynthesen oder Operationen am Knochen. Unfallheilkd 83:226
41. Rehn J, Lies A (1981) Die Pathogenese der Pseudarthrose, ihre Diagnostik und Therapie. Unfallheilkd 85:1
42. Rhinelander FW (1974) Tibial blood supply in relation to fracture healing. Clin Orthop 105:34
43. Rhinelander FW (1980) Vascular proliferation and blood supply during fracture healing. In: Upthoff HK (ed) Current concepts of internal fixation of fractures. Springer, Berlin Heidelberg New York
44. Rittmann WW, Matter P (1977) Die offene Fraktur. Huber, Bern Stuttgart Wien
45. Rüedi Th, Webb JK, Allgöwer M (1976) Experience with the dynamic compression plate (DCP) in 418 recent fractures of the tibial shaft. Injury 7:252
46. Rüter A, Kuck W, Burri C (1978) Dorsale Plattenosteosynthese an der Tibia. 42. Jahrestag Dtsch Ges Unfallheilkd 23.–25. Nov., Berlin
47. Schlenzka R, Gotzen L, Warmbild M (1982) Stabilitätsunterschungen an einem ventralen Klammerfixateur der Tibia. Teil II: Biegebelastung. Unfallheilkd (im Druck)
48. Schweiberer L, Dambe LT, Eitel F, Klapp F (1974) Revascularisation der Tibia nach konservativer und operativer Frakturenbehandlung. Hefte Unfallheilkd 119:18
49. Schweiberer L, Klapp F, Chevalier H (1975) Platten und Schraubenosteosynthese bei Frakturen und Pseudarthrosen des Ober- und Unterschenkels. Chirurg 46:155
50. Sisk DT (1981) Fractures. In: Campbells Operative Orthopaedics. Mosby, St. Louis
51. Smith JEM (1974) Results of early and delayed internal fixation for tibial shaft fractures. A review of 470 fractures. J Bone Joint Surg 56B:469
52. Stürmer KM, Schuchardt W (1980) Neue Aspekte der gedeckten Marknagelung und des Aufbohrens der Markhöhle im Tierexperiment. III. Knochenheilung. Gefäßversorgung und Knochenumbau. Unfallheilkd 83:433
53. Szyskowitz R, Reschauer R, Seggl W (1981) Gefahren der Plattenosteosynthese und Möglichkeiten des Fixateur externe in der Frakturerstversorgung. Hefte Unfallheilkd 153:179
54. Thunold J, Varhaug JE, Bjerkeset T (1976) Tibial shaft fractures treated with rigid internal fixation. Injury 7:125
55. Trueta J (1974) Blood supply and the rate of healing of tibial fractures. Clin Orthop 105:11

56. Tscherne H (1975) Die Behandlung der offenen Frakturen. Tagungsbericht 10. Unfallseminar, Hannover
57. Tscherne H, Brüggemann H (1976) Die Weichteilbehandlung bei Osteosynthesen, insbesondere bei offenen Frakturen. Unfallheilkd 79:467
58. Warmbold M, Gotzen L, Schlenzka R (1982) Stabilitätsunterschungen an einem ventralen Klammerfixateur der Tibia. Teil I: Axiale Belastung. Unfallheilkd (im Druck)
59. Weiß H, Wissing H, Schmit-Neuerburg KP (1978) Komplikationsrate und Infektrisiko offener und geschlossener Unterschenkelbrüche mit Weichteilschaden. Akt Traumatol 8:329
60. Weller S (1981) Biomechanische Prinzipien in der operativen Knochenbruchbehandlung. Akt Traumatol 11:195
61. Weller S (1982) Der Fixateur externe im Dienst der Prophylaxe und Therapie von Infektionen. Akt Traumatol 12:43
62. Widenfalk B, Ponton B, Karlström G (1979) Open fractures of the shaft of the tibia: analysis of wound and fracture treatment. Injury 11:36
63. Willenegger H (1972) Licht und Schatten über der Indikation zur Knochenbruchbehandlung. Mschr Unfallheilkd 75:455

Compartment Syndrome: Etiology, Pathophysiology, Anatomy, Localization, Diagnosis and Treatment

V. Echtermeyer, H. Tscherne, H.-J. Oestern and E. van der Zypen

1. Introduction

Considering the prevalence and great clinical importance of the compartment syndromes, it is remarkable how few physicians are well versed in their signs and symptoms, and how often these conditions are overlooked or misinterpreted. After thrombosis, compartment syndromes are the most frequent complication of bone fractures, especially those involving the tibia. Functional deficits that arise during fracture treatment may be distributed largely to the development of unrecognized compartment syndromes (Tscherne 1982).

Today we can define the compartment syndrome in fairly accurate terms: It is a condition in which an increase of tissue pressure within a closed space impedes the blood supply and function of the tissues containing within that space. This definition encompasses the four factors necessary for a compartment syndrome to occur: A *closed space* in which *increased tissue pressure* causes a *diminished blood flow to the tissues,* leading to *disturbances of neuromuscular function* (Matsen III 1980. Mubarak, Hargens 1981).

2. Etiology

Two factors are essential to the pathogenesis of a compartment syndrome:
a) An envelope which encloses a circumscribed space.
b) An increase of tissue pressure within that envelope.

The first factor, an enclosed envelope, may be the epimysium, an osseofibrous sheath like that in the anterior tibial compartment, or the fascia alone, as in the gluteal compartment. In addition, the skin or a constricting dressing may create a limiting boundary.

The second factor, an elevated tissue pressure, may be caused either by compression from without or by an increase in the volume of the compartmental contents.

Initially, an increase in compartmental contents is associated with only a slight rise of intracompartmental pressure, apparently owing to the large compliance of the investing fascia. But as the volume of the contents continues to expand, the pressure within the compartment begins to rise exponentially. This is confirmed by the experiments of Whitesides (1971), who found that when the contents of the anterior tibial compartment were increased in volume from 110% to 140%, the intracompartmental pressure rose by only 30%. However, an additional 30% increase from 150% to 180% caused the pressure to increase by 75 mmHg (from 45 to 120 mmHg).

The volume of the compartmental contents may be increased by hemorrhage, perivascular infusions, or by fluid losses due to abnormal capillary permeability in the way of prolonged ischemia. If the circulation subsequently returns to normal, there will be a heavy extravasation from the damaged capillaries. This post-ischemic swelling has been analyzed quantitatively in experimental studies. Fuhrman and Crismon (1951) measured the water content of rabbit muscles two hours after varying periods of tourniquet ischemia. They found that 3 hours' ischemia increased post-ischemic swelling by 30%–60%.

The size of the compartment may be decreased by the surgical closure of fascial defects or by excessive limb traction in the treatment of fractures.

There are certain predisposing injuries which greatly increase the risk for developing a compartment syndrome. Thus, it is possible to make a distinction between low-risk and high-risk injuries. Primarily healthy trauma patients who have no shock-induced peripheral hypoxia are assigned to the low-risk group. These patients have simple fracture configurations caused by an indirect mechanism, and they have no concomitant injuries. Skiing fractures are a typical example.

Foremost among the high-risk factors are vascular injuries with peripheral ischemia. High-energy traumata are another frequent cause of compartment syndromes. Grade II and grade III soft tissue injuries, especially those associated with closed fractures, and "bumper" injuries causing a segmental fracture of the tibia constitute typical high-risk situations. Comminuted fractures of the distal tibia also belong to the high-risk category. Moreover, all multiply injured patients are predisposed to compartment syndromes on account of their reduced peripheral flow.

3. Pathophysiology of Compartment Syndromes

Normal tissue function is ensured by a circulation which is sufficient to meet the metabolic demands of the tissue. In compartment syndromes, the blood supply to the tissue is compromised to a point where it can no longer satisfy these demands, and functional deficits arise.

There is general agreement that the blood flow to the muscles is determined not so much by the absolute pressure within the fascial compartment as by the relationship between the intracompartmental pressure and the blood pressure. This is especially true in multiply injured patients, who are predisposed to compartmental syndromes by their decreased peripheral flow. In experiments by Zweifach et al. (1964), an intracompartmental pressure of 25 mmHg in animals with systemic hypotension produced the same effects as a pressure of 40–50 mmHg in normotensive animals.

There is diversity of opinion as to the mechanism responsible for the decline in tissue perfusion. Several theories have been proposed:

Arterial Spasm Theory

Foisie (1942), Benjamin (1957), Gardner (1970) and Eaton and Green (1972) theorize that the increased tissue pressure induces an arterial spasm which in turn is responsible for intracompartmental ischemia. However, the presence of pulses distal to the affected compartment would seem to contradict this explanation. Moreover, arteriograms in patients with compartment syndromes tend to show a gradual narrowing of the blood vessels as they traverse the affected compartment – a finding which is not characteristic of arterial spasm.

Critical Closing Pressure Theory

Burton (1951) and later Ashton (1975) observed that when large external pressures are applied to an extremity, the blood flow ceases before the difference between the mean arterial pressure and applied pressure is zero. These observations led to speculations on the existence of a "critical closing pressure." According to this theory, a significant transmural pressure difference (mean arterial pressure minus tissue pressure) is required to keep the arterioles patent. If tissue pressure becomes so high that the transmural pressure is insufficient, the arterioles will actively close, and blood flow will cease. Attempts to determine a critical closing pressure have been made almost exclusively at a normal venous pressure (Burton 1951; Ashton 1975).

Arteriovenous Gradient Theory

This theory holds that increases in tissue pressure lower the local arteriovenous gradient, producing a decrease in local blood flow. A reduction of perfusion below the level needed to meet metabolic demands results in the functional disturbances characteristic of compartment syndrome.

The relationship between the arteriovenous gradient and local perfusion is defined by the equation $LBF = P_A - P_V/R$ (Feigl 1974), where LBF is the local blood flow, P_A is the local arterial pressure, P_V is the local venous pressure, and R is local vascular resistance. Because the veins have collapsible walls, the pressure within them (P_V) cannot be less than the ambient tissue pressure (P_T). It follows, then, that as the tissue pressure increases, the local venous pressure must also rise (Lanz 1979). The increased local venous pressure has the effect of lowering the local arteriovenous gradient. This phenomenon has been confirmed by direct measurements of local venous pressure (Ryder et al. 1943; Kjellmer 1964; Matsen et al. 1980).

Some reduction of the local arteriovenous gradient can be compensated for by a change in local vascular resistance. This mechanism, known as autoregulation, can keep local perfusion at adequate levels over a fairly wide arteriovenous gradient (Feigl 1974). But if this gradient becomes significantly reduced, autoregulation is no longer effective. At this point local perfusion is determined essentially by the local arteriovenous gradient. As tissue pressure continues to rise, local perfusion becomes unable to meet tissue demands, and functional deficits occur.

This theory is particularly useful from a clinical standpoint, for it implies that a decrease in the local arterial pressure (e.g. by elevating the leg above the level of the heart) will amplify the circulatory effects of an increased tissue pressure. The theory further implies that reducing the local venous pressure through tissue decompression is an effective means of restoring tissue perfusion in the face of an impending compartment syndrome. Finally, this theory explains the preservation of the pulses and distal circulation that is frequently observed in the presence of compartment syndromes. The pulses and distal circulation may remain for two reasons: First, the increase in tissue pressure that generally occurs in compartment syndromes has little effect on the arterial flow. Second, the venous pressure in the fingers or toes distal to the compartment is usually normal, resulting in a normal distal arteriovenous gradient and digital blood flow.

4. Anatomy and Localization

A compartment syndrome can develop in any region where muscles, blood vessels and nerves are enclosed within relatively unyielding compartments. The muscles within a compartment represent a functional unit. The overlying fascia may serve as the origin of the muscles, being adherent to them and forming a unit with the epimysium. In most cases, however, the fascia and epimysium are separate from each other. This enables the fascia to serve as an abutment for the muscle, increasing its mechanical efficiency by about 15% (Garfin et al. 1981).

Compartments of the Upper Extremity

The deltoid muscle lies within a powerful fascial compartment which generally is divided into two distinct subcompartments by an intermuscular septum. The lateral subcompartment is traversed by the axillary nerve and the posterior humeral circumflex artery. The deep fascia of the deltoid muscle separates these structures from the lateral head of the triceps muscle, which covers the radial nerve canal. The long head of the triceps has its own thick fascial sheath which merges distally with the common extensor compartment. The fascial sheath of the coracobrachialis muscle is likewise incomplete and blends distally with the flexor compartment of the forearm. Thus, four fascial compartments can be distinguished in the region of the shoulder girdle: two for the deltoid muscle, one partially enclosed extensor compartment, and one incompletely septated flexor compartment.

The main compartment of the deltoid muscle extends distally to the mid-upper arm. The neurovascular structures of the common extensor compartment run along the shaft of the humerus as they traverse the radial nerve canal. The flexor compartment shows an incomplete septation in the mid-upper arm. The septum accompanies the musculocutaneous nerve between the brachialis and biceps brachii muscles (Fig. 1).

The forearm contains more closed compartments than was previously recognized. Ten completely isolated muscle compartments can be identified. There are four compartments on the dorsal side, the compartments of the superficial and deep extensors being framed by the compartments of extensor carpi radialis and extensor carpi ulnaris. The deep extensor compartment is probably the most important, because the muscles there (abductor pollicis longus, extensor pollicis brevis and longus, extensor indicis proprius) are contained within an extremely firm compartment bounded deeply by the ulna, radius and interosseus membrane. If possible, this compartment should not be opened proximally due to its unfavourable relation to the other compartments.

On the volar side, flexor digitorum superficialis and flexor digitorum profundus each possessses its own fascial compartment. The superficial flexor compartment is surrounded by the compartments of flexor carpi ulnaris and flexor carpi radialis. The pronator teres and brachioradialis muscles also have their own fascial compartments. The ulnar compartments are always held under some degree of tension by the firm bicipital aponeurosis. This can lead to a rapid constriction of the ulnar veins and interosseous vein when a compartment syndrome develops. The bicipital aponeurosis also exerts tension on the ulnar and radial arteries and their accompanying veins, as well as on the median nerve, which traverses the fascial compartment of pronator teres before entering the compartment of

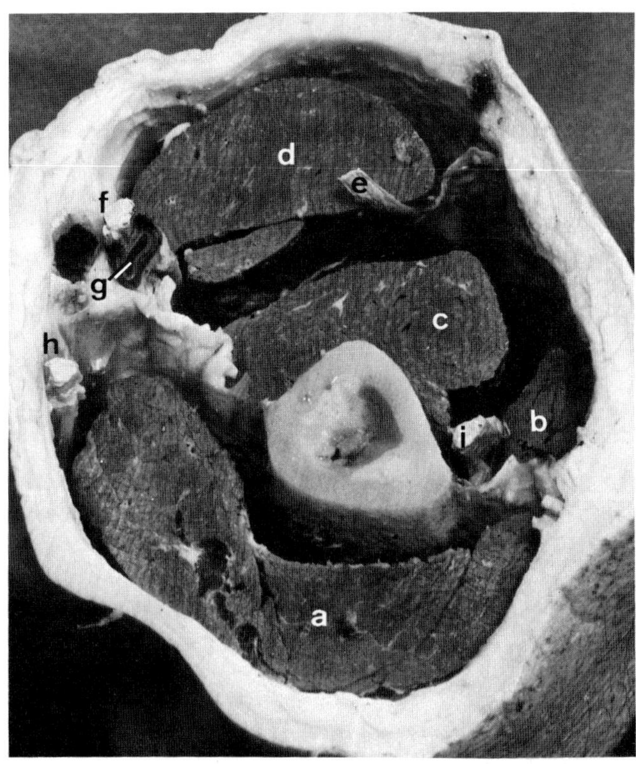

Fig. 1. Transverse section through the distal portion of the right upper arm, proximal aspect. *a* = extensor compartment; *b* = brachioradialis muscle; *c* = brachialis muscle; *d* = biceps muscle; *e* = lateral antebrachial cutaneous nerve; *f* = median nerve; *g* = brachial artery and vein; *h* = ulnar nerve; *i* = radial nerve

flexor digitorum superficialis. Thus, surgical division of the bicipital aponeurosis effects a significant decompression of neurovascular structures in the proximal forearm (Fig. 2).

In the distal third of the forearm, the extensor compartment undergoes a marked change. The superficial extensor compartment in this region is extremely thin and narrow. The fascial compartments of extensor carpi ulnaris and extensor carpi radialis also become narrower. On the radial side, the deep extensor compartment becomes superficial and is readily accessible to surgical decompression.

The hand contains the fascial compartments of the interosseous muscles. The palmar and dorsal interosseous muscles for each finger are enclosed within fascial sheaths which are divided from one another by septa. Thus, seven interosseous compartments may be distinguished. It is important to note that the fascial compartment of adductor pollicis can be reached from the dorsal side between the index and middle fingers.

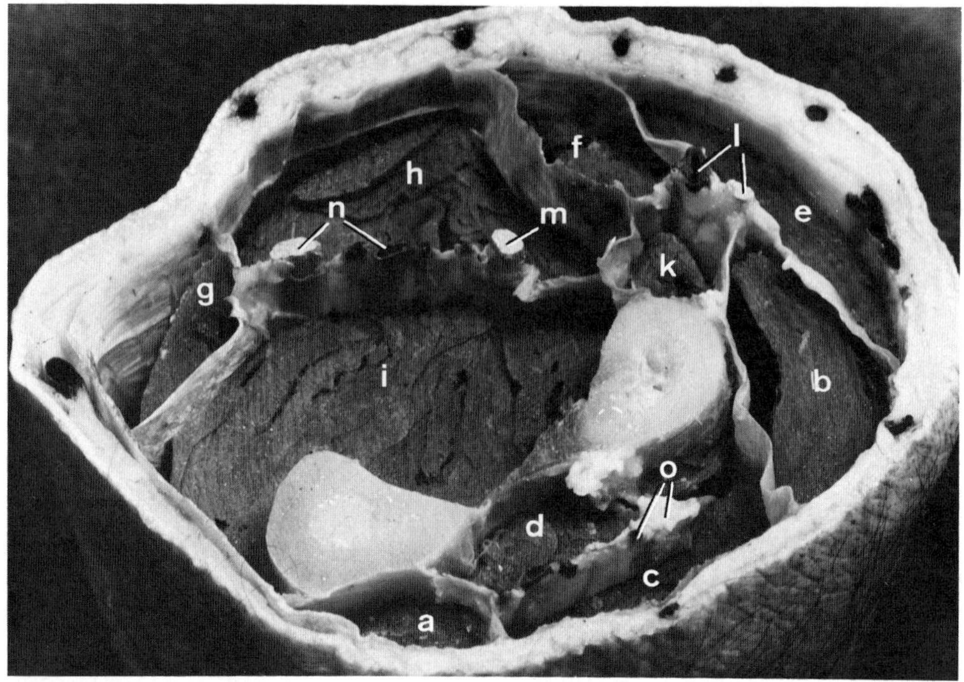

Fig. 2. Transverse section through the proximal third of the right forearm, proximal aspect. Two closed fascial compartments can be identified. *a* = extensor digiti minimi muscle; *b* = extensor carpi radialis muscle; *c* = superficial extensor; *d* = deep extensor compartment; *e* = brachioradialis muscle; *f* = flexor carpi radialis muscle; *g* = flexor carpi ulnaris muscle; *h* = superficial flexors; *i* = deep flexors; *k* = pronator teres muscle; *l* = superficial branch of radial nerve and radial artery; *m* = median nerve; *n* = ulnar nerve and artery; *o* = deep branch of radial nerve with posterior interosseus vein and artery

Compartments of the Lower Extremity

The gluteal region contains three compartments: one enclosing the gluteus maximus, a common compartment containing gluteus medius and minimus, and one enclosing tensor fasciae latae. The latter is the strongest compartment in the human body.

The tensor fasciae latae compartment is one of seven fascial compartments which can be distinguished in the proximal thigh (Fig. 3). The sciatic nerve lies in a septum which divides the ischiocrural muscles from the adductors. The adductors are contained within three compartments, sartorius and adductor longus each occupying a closed fascial compartment, and adductor brevis and adductor magnus occupying a common, incompletely septated fascial compartment. The fully enclosed compartment of sartorius serves to isolate this muscle from the extensors of the quadriceps group. The quadriceps muscle bellies occupy a common fascial compartment, although the individual parts of the quadriceps muscle are separated from one another by incomplete septa which carry blood vessels through that region. The septa of the extensor compartment disappear at the junction of the middle and distal thirds of the thigh, giving rise to a common extensor compartment

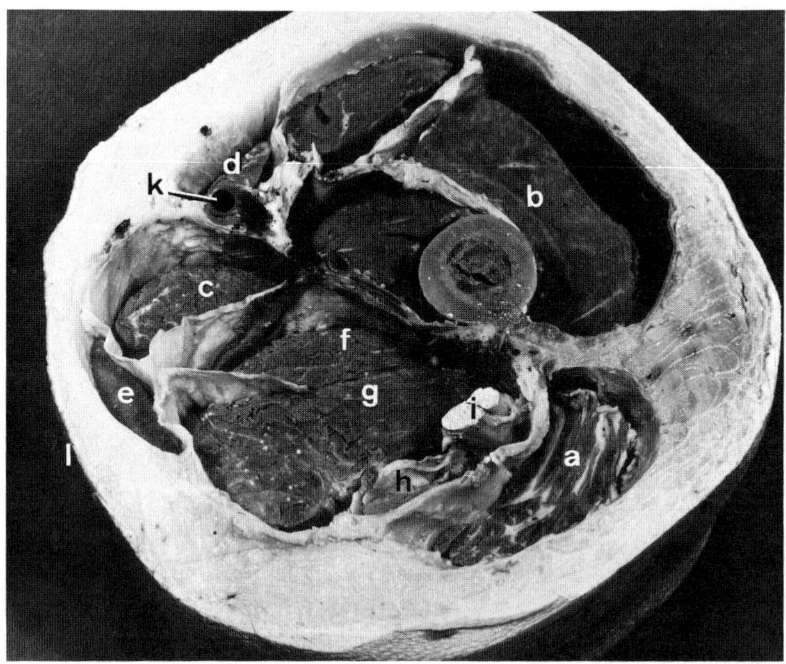

Fig. 3. Transverse section through the proximal part of the right thigh, proximal aspect. Seven compartments exist in this region. *a* = tensor fasciae latae muscle; *b* = quadriceps muscle; *c* = adductor longus muscle; *d* = sartorius muscle; *e* = gracilis muscle; *f* = adductor brevis muscle; *g* = adductor magnus muscle; *h* = semimembranosus muscle; *i* = sciatic nerve; *k* = femoral artery and vein

that is readily accessible from the lateral side. The sartorius muscle courses medially in its closed fascial sheath, coming in close contact with the gracilis compartment. A medial incision which starts at the junction of the middle and distal thirds of the thigh and is carried distally over the sartorius can be used to open the adductor compartment, extensor compartment, sartorius compartment and gracilis compartment. The adductor longus compartment can additionally be opened by extending the incision proximally.

With regard to the flexor compartment, one anatomic peculiarity should be noted. While the semitendinosus muscle possesses its own, firm fascial envelope the fascial compartment of biceps femoris communicates openly with the fascial compartment of semimembranosus immediately below the fascia lata. Thus, a sagittal incision over the flexor muscles will simultaneously open the compartments of the biceps and semimembranosus muscles while also exposing the fascial compartment of the semitendinosus, which can then be opened with a second incision.

In the distal part of the thigh, the femoral artery and vein course posteriorally in the vastoadductor canal. The vastoadductor membrane separates the vessels from the terminal division of the sciatic nerve. This bifurcation is flanked by the communicating compartments of the biceps femoris laterally and the semimembranosus medially. If it becomes necessary to decompress the vessels in the vastoadductor canal, access is most readily gained at the lateral intermuscular septum, i.e., between the quadriceps and biceps muscles.

The lower leg contains four well-known fascial compartments whose size vary considerably in a proximal-to-distal direction. Two compartments are of particular clinical importance: the extensor compartment and the deep flexor compartment. Both compartments are bounded by the tibia, fibula and interosseous membrane, and both are traversed by a major neurovascular bundle of the lower leg: the deep peroneal nerve accompanied by the

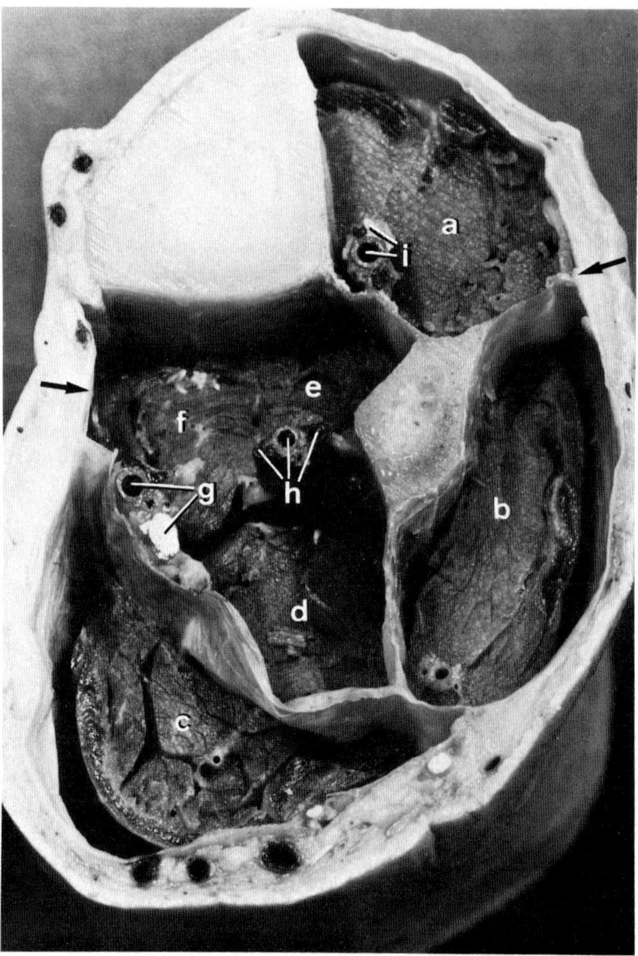

Fig. 4. Transverse section through the distal part of the right lower leg, proximal aspect. The extensor compartment (*a*) and peroneus compartment (*b*) are accessible through a single incision (*arrow*). The deep flexor compartment [flexor digitorum longus (*f*), tibialis posterior (*e*), flexor hallucis longus (*d*)] directly underlies superficial fascia at the posterior tibial border in the distal third of the lower leg (*arrow*), where it can be safely decompressed. *c* = triceps surae muscle; *g* posterior tibial artery and tibial nerve; *h* = peroneal artery and veins; *i* = anterior tibial artery and deep peroneal nerve

anterior tibial artery and veins in the extensor compartment, and the tibial nerve, posterior tibial artery, peroneal artery and four accompanying veins in the deep flexor compartment. The peroneus muscle also occupies a closed fascial compartment, which is separated from the flexor compartment by the powerful lateral intermuscular septum. The superficial peroneal nerve which traverses this compartment is not accompanied by major vessels. The gastrocnemius and soleus muscles form the principal bulk of the proximal lower leg. The narrow, deep flexor compartment should not be opened proximally; this compartment becomes larger distally at the expense of the superficial flexor compartment (Fig. 4).

In the plantar region of the foot, four groups of compartments can be identified. There is one septated compartment each for the muscles of the great toe and small toe, and one compartment for the long and short digital flexors. These three plantar compartments intercommunicate distally. The fourth group of compartments enclose the interosseous muscles. As in the hand, these compartments are accessible from the dorsal side.

5. Diagnosis of Compartment Syndromes

a) Clinical Examination. In the conscious patient, the earliest and most important symptom is a burning, boring pain of acute onset which may be spasmodic in nature and tends to increase with time. Sensory aberrations are also reported in the form of paresthesias, hypoesthesias, and rapid sensory losses. In cooperative patients, disturbances of muscular function are demonstrable as motor weakness after 2–4 hours' ischemia. On palpation, the affected muscles are tender and have a firm to stony-hard consistency. Peripheral arterial pulses and capillary perfusion are intact in the early stage, provided there is not concomitant arterial injury (Fig. 5).

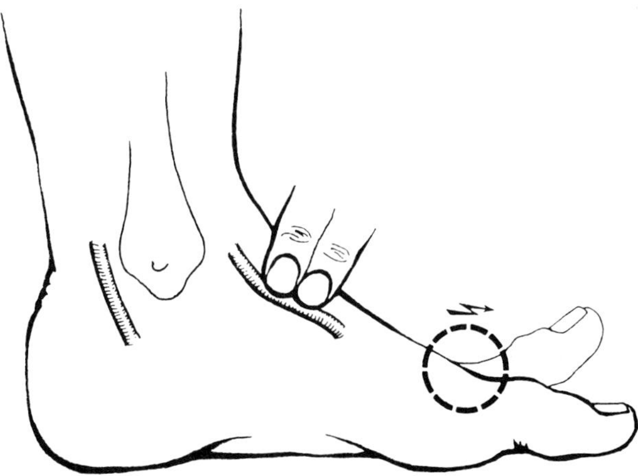

Fig. 5. Symptoms of the frequent anterior tibial compartment syndrome with paresthesias of the first web space and weak dorsiflexion of the great toe. Despite the impaired microcirculation, the peripheral pulses are often intact

b) Measurement of Tissue Pressure. The most useful adjunctive technique for diagnosing a compartmental syndrome in unconscious patients is the measurement of subfascial tissue pressure, which normally ranges between 0 and 5 mmHg. The microcirculation ceases when the difference between the subfascial pressure and diastolic blood pressure falls below 30 mmHg. In normotensive patients, however, even absolute pressure levels of 30–40 mmHg should be cause for alarm (Wissing 1980; Mubarak et al. 1981). While a transitory pressure rise of up to 40 mmHg can usually be tolerated without permanent injury, sustained pressures of 60 mmHg or more will always produce irreversible changes.

Whitesides (1975) has devised a relatively simple technique for measuring tissue pressure. The technique employs a mercury manometer, a syringe, and a cannula interconnected by means of a 3-way stopcock. As the plunger of the air-filled syringe is depressed, the manometer will indicate the pressure required to inject a small amount of saline from the cannula into the muscle compartment. This reading will equal the subfascial tissue pressure in mmHg.

Mubarak (1978) and Matsen (1980) have developed similar techniques employing indwelling catheters. An infusion rate of 0.7 cm^3 per day is used for continuous pressure monitoring. Experiments have shown that the measured pressure is relatively independent of the infusion rate. An acute 40-fold increase of the infusion rate from 0.7 to 28 cm^3 per day produces only a 4-mmHg increase in the measured pressure. Hargens (1978) found that the acute infusion of 2 cm^3 plasma into the anterolateral compartment of the dog (volume 40 cm^3) raised intracompartmental pressure from 30 to 45 mmHg.

A pressure increase caused by infusion of saline is unlikely to be a problem, however, for several reasons:

1. Saline or Ringer's lactate is absorbed 3 times more rapidly than plasma.
2. Three days of pressure monitoring would be required to infuse a volume of 2 cm^3 into the compartment.
3. Compartments in humans are more than 10 times larger than the canine anterolateral compartment.

We use a measuring system which employs a large-gauge cannula having three extra perforations near the tip (Fig. 6a). It is connected to a fluid-filled infusion system which enables the interstitial tissue pressure to be read from a scale, similar to the measurement of central venous pressure (Fig. 6b). The saline-filled cannula is introduced over a needle into the compartment to be measured, as in a venipuncture. The needle is then withdrawn while injecting a small amount of NaCl to ensure that the cannula is fluid-filled. The scale is zeroed by adjusting a horizontal slide, and NcCl-filled infusion tubing is connected to the cannula and syringe via a 3-way stopcock. The fluid meniscus in the tubing is initially set at 20 mmHg. By watching the meniscus, it can be determined whether an elevated tissue pressure is present. If the meniscus does not fall, NaCl is infused via the stopcock in 10-mmHg increments until a fall in the meniscus is noted. Five minutes are then allowed for the system to equilibrate so that the infused saline will not cause falsely high values. The volume of fluid infused is negligible compared to the volume of the human compartment, for comparisons of pressure measured with a transducer and monitor have shown no differences in values measured over the range from 30 mmHg to 100 mmHg. In the normal and slightly elevated range (< 30 mmHg), the readings from a water manometer are slightly higher (1–2 mmHg) than those obtained with a Statham element.

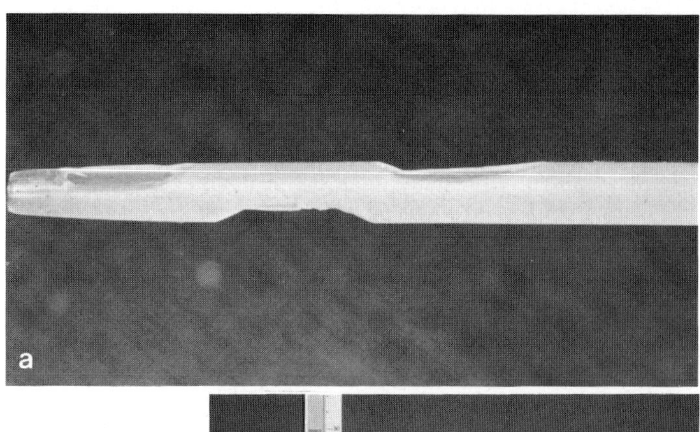

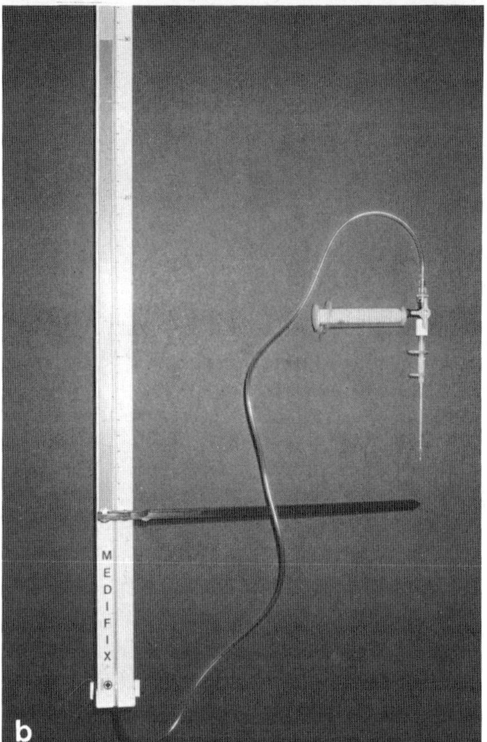

Fig. 6. a Plastic cannula with three elliptical perforations at its tip for use in the measurement of intracompartmental pressures. **b** Overall view of the measuring system

The following criteria serve to confirm patency of the system:

1. Digital tissue compression near the cannula tip causes a sudden and reversible pressure rise.
2. Active muscle contraction also causes a pressure rise, which regresses on relaxation.
3. In the pathologic range (> 40 mmHg), the fluid meniscus fluctuates in synchrony with the pulse.

c) Blood Flow Measurements. Doppler ultrasonography is very useful in identifying sites of arterial stenosis or occlusion. The study is simple to perform, objective and noninvasive.

In extremital injuries, its main role is to exclude or confirm the presence of concomitant arterial lesions.

The same is true of arteriography, which is indicated if pulses are absent or diminished, or if peripheral ischemia is noted. A narrowing of peripheral arteries without other vascular pathology should be viewed simply as a consequence of ischemic muscle swelling. A normal arteriogram does not exclude a coexisting compartmental syndrome.

Phlebography is of value in differentiating a venous thrombosis from a compartment syndrome, as well as in demonstrating a chronic compartment syndrome caused by sustained overexertion of the tibialis anterior (Renemann 1975).

6. Differential Diagnosis

It is frequently difficult to differentiate a compartment syndrome from post-traumatic pain and from primary neural or vascular injuries (Wissing, Schmit-Neuerburg 1982). Exclusion must be made from:

1. Acute phlebothrombosis and thrombophlebitis, in which the standard venous pressure points on the extremities are highly sensitive.
2. Acute nerve paralyses. These lesions have a sudden onset and, unlike compartment syndromes, are unaccompanied by swelling and muscle pain on passive stretching. Traumatic and ischemic pareses can be differentiated by electrical stimulation of the motor nerve trunk (Matsen et al. 1980).
3. Infections are always associated with systemic signs of inflammation.
4. In rare cases drugs containing ergotamine can produce a clinical picture of ergotism, characterized by sudden ischemic pain resulting from arterial spasms. The spasms are relieved by nitroglycerine and by the ganglion blockade produced by peridural anesthesia.

7. Classification of Compartment Syndromes

A compartment syndrome may be classified as *impending* or *frank* by the severity of its clinical signs (Echtermeyer et al. 1982). With an impending compartment syndrome, peripheral blood flow is not yet diminished, and neurologic deficits are absent or mild. A cardinal feature is pain that is out of proportion to the primary injury. Pressures measured in the fascial compartments are in the high-normal range. 30–40 mmHg has been empirically defined as the critical pressure level (Matsen et al. 1976; Mubarak et al. 1978; Owen et al. 1978; Akeson et al. 1981), though this can vary considerably in patients with peripheral vascular disease and post-traumatic shock.

In frank compartment syndrome a significant neurologic deficit has already developed, and disturbances of blood flow are apparent.

The indication for surgical decompression is based essentially upon clinical symptoms and measurements of tissue pressure. The normal subfascial pressure is less than 10 mm Hg. Pressures between 20 and 30 mm Hg are not yet an indication for decompression, but the patient should be closely observed. If the subfascial tissue pressure rises to between 30 and 40 mm Hg, surgical decompression is performed if a neuromuscular deficit is present. If pressures rise above 40 mm Hg, a decompressive dermatofasciotomy is urgently indicated.

8. General Primary Treatment

When a compartment syndrome is suspected, the most important immediate measure is the wide splitting of any constricting dressing that have been applied. As Garfin (1981) showed experimentally, the wide spreading of a plaster cast reduces the subfascial pressure in the anterior tibial compartment by 30%. Removal of the cast can reduce pressure to 15% of the initial value. Overinflated anti-shock splints can produce a constricting action similar to that of plaster casts.

The extreme elevation of an extremity decreases the arteriovenous pressure difference (Fig. 7). The results of the diminished arterial flow are hypoxia and acidosis in the injured limb. Thus, a useful preventive measure is either to avoid elevating the extremity, or to elevate it no more than 10 cm above the level of the atria. In critically injured patients, aggressive volume replacement aimed at raising the mean arterial pressure is vital for improving the arteriovenous gradient and preventing compartment syndrome. General hypotension tends to accelerate ischemic damage to muscles and nerves, and so lower intracompartmental pressures are needed to produce neuromuscular deficits in hypotensive individuals (Matsen et al. 1980; Zweifach et al. 1980).

Vasodilators and sympathicolytic drugs are of no benefit in compartment syndromes. The only effective treatment is causal: surgical decompression to reduce the intracompartmental pressure.

9. General Operative Technique

To minimize the duration of muscle ischemia, the operation is performed without a tourniquet. On completion of the decompressive procedure, the viability of the intracompartmental muscles is assessed. The best criteria for muscle viability are the "4 C's": contractil-

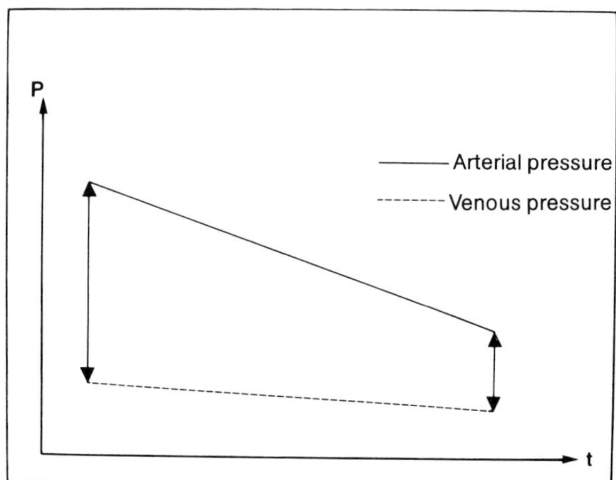

Fig. 7. Reduction of the intracompartmental arteriovenous pressure difference by elevation of the extremity

ity, consistency, color, and capacity to bleed. Healthy muscle contracts when touched, has a normal consistency, is reddish-brown or slightly livid in color, and bleeds when cut.

In patients with an impending compartment syndrome, a prophylactic fasciotomy is performed if operations have been planned which will heighten the risk of compartment ischemia. This includes procedures such as bone grafting and compression plating of the femur, which would tend to increase the contents of the compartment. Prophylactic fasciotomy is also indicated when compartmental contents are constricted, e.g., by a bone-lengthening internal or external fixation of the lower extremity.

If operative stabilization of a long bone is not planned, we do not feel that a prophylactic fasciotomy is necessary under low-risk conditions. However, the patient should be kept under close clinical observation, and subfascial tissue pressure should be closely monitored.

When a frank compartment syndrome is present, a *therapeutic dermatofasciotomy* is performed by incising the fascia longitudinally and transversely. The decompressed muscles are inspected, and devitalized portions and clotted blood are removed. The viability criteria listed above will guide the surgeon in determining the necessary extent of the debridement. If signs are inconclusive, it is better not to resect, for the regenerative capacity of the muscles often cannot be foreseen at operation. When the patient is later returned to the operating room for skin closure, a second look can be taken and the need for further debridement assessed. In frank compartment syndrome the wound is not closed primarily, but is simply covered with a synthetic skin dressing. Primary wound closure carries a high risk of rebound compartment syndrome (Fig. 8), as the post-ischemic swelling that occurs 6–12 hours postoperatively leads to a renewed increase in muscle volume (Matsen 1980).

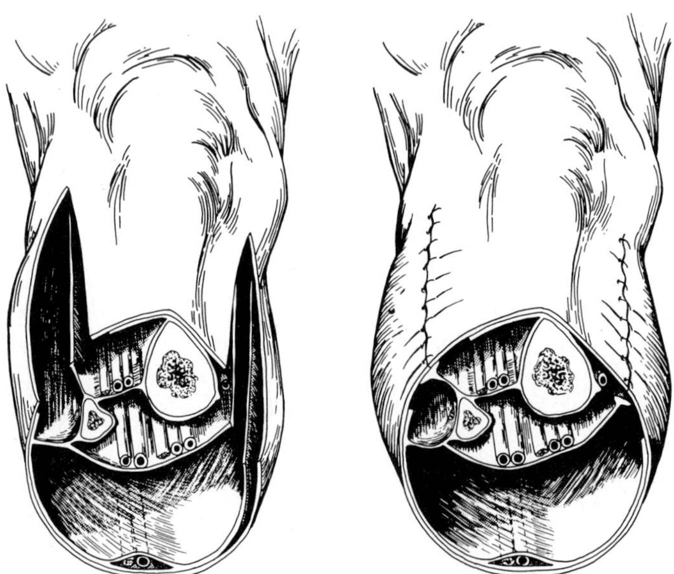

Fig. 8a, b. Development of a rebound compartment syndrome. **a** Condition following a four-compartment double-incision fasciotomy. **b** Primary skin closure can induce a rebound compartment syndrome 6–12 hours later as a result of post-schemic muscle swelling

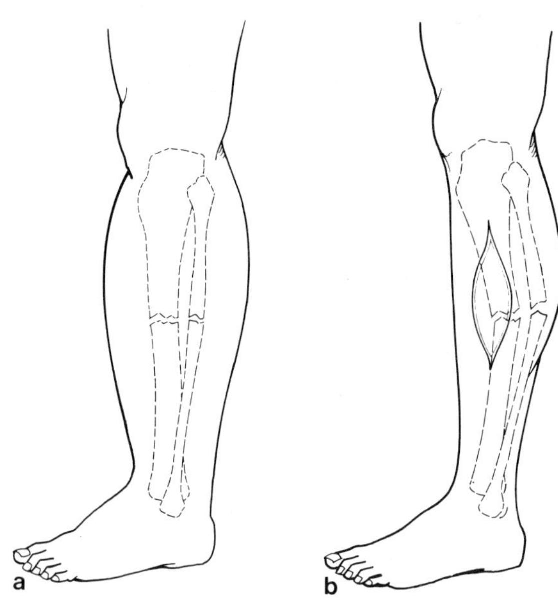

Fig. 9. a When a compartment syndrome accompanies a fracture, the tense, swollen soft tissues tend to exert a splinting action on the fractured bone. **b** Fracture stability is reduced when the tissues are surgically decompressed

After decompression has been carried out, a stable operative fixation of the accompanying fracture should be undertaken for two reasons (Fig. 9):

1. The fasciotomy destabilizes the fracture.
2. The fasciotomy converts a primarily closed fracture into a secondarily open one that is susceptible to infection.

10. Techniques of Surgical Decompression

The following incisions have proved useful for the surgical decompression of compartments:

In the *shoulder region,* the deltoid muscle compartment is approached through a slightly curved incision which starts below the clavicle at the level of the coracoid process and passes caudally, following the line of the infraclavicular fossa. Because the muscle is subdivided by multiple septa, a fasciotomy in this region should be supplemented by an epimysiotomy. In the *upper arm,* the approach for decompressing the anterior or posterior compartment depends upon the nature of concomitant injuries. In the presence of vascular lesions, a medial incision is indicated (Fig. 10). If internal fixation of the humerus is proposed, a lateral approach is used.

The volar compartment of the *forearm* is approached through a volar-ulnar incision. It is important to divide the inelastic bicipital aponeurosis (Fig. 11), which, together with the pronator teres muscle and biceps tendon, forms a V-shaped aperture through which pass the brachial artery and median nerve. The compartment containing the superficial flexors

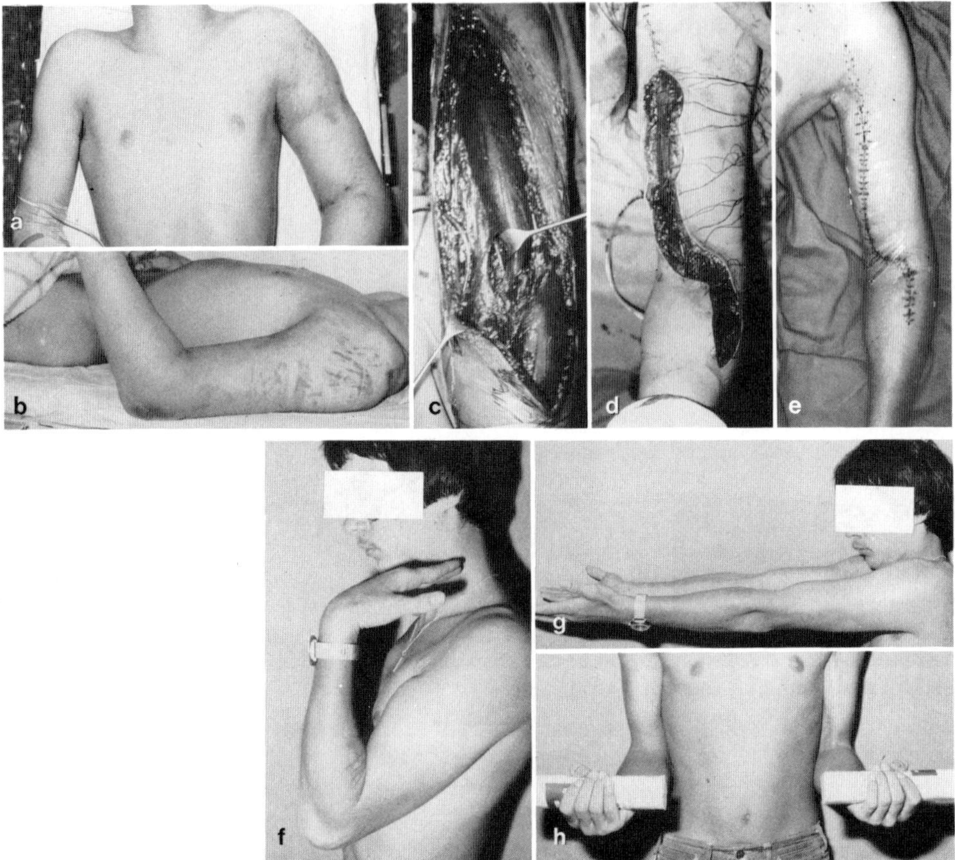

Fig. 10. a, b A compartment syndrome developed in this patient whose left shoulder and left upper arm were caught beneath the wheel of an automobile. No osseous injuries were sustained. c Appearance of the arm following surgical decompression. d Partial skin closure and preplacement of sutures. e Secondary suture of residual defect. f–h Function one year postinjury

is opened over the flexor carpi ulnaris muscle. The deep compartment can be reached by ulnarward retraction of this muscle. When releasing the deep flexor muscles, care is taken not to injure the ulnar neurovascular bundle. Distally the transverse carpal ligament should also be divided. Release of the extensor muscles is effected simply by incising the antebrachial fascia on the radial side.

In the *hand,* a compartment syndrome of the interosseous muscles was described by Finochietto as early as 1920. The interosseous compartments of the long fingers are decompressed from the dorsal side by the technique of Buck-Gramcko (1974), in which a longitudinal or slightly curved skin incision is made over the 2nd or 4th metacarpal bone, as needed, to reach the adjacent interosseous compartment. The thenar and hypothenar compartments are decompressed from the volar side. The carpal tunnel and retinaculum,

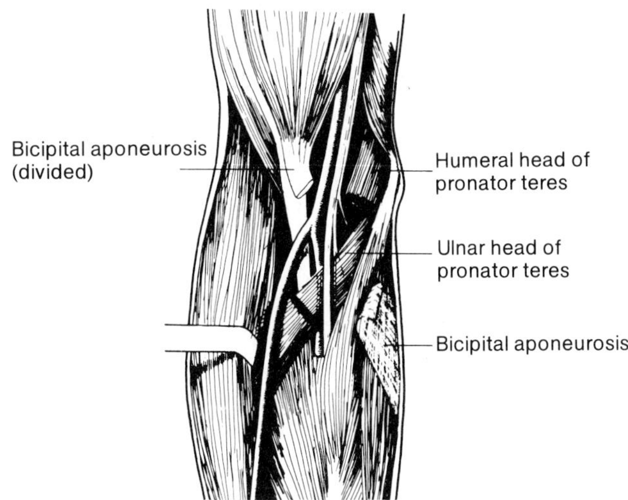

Fig. 11. Schematic drawing of the volar surface of the elbow following division of the bicipital aponeurosis and partial resection of the humeral head of pronator teres

together with Guyon's canal, are opened by an S-shaped palmar incision. Great care should be taken to spare the thenar motor branch of the median nerve.

In decompressing the *gluteal muscles,* the incision may be made just distal and parallel to the iliac crest, or it may correspond to the standard posterior approach to the hip joint (Fig. 12). Both a fasciotomy and epimysiotomy are required to decompress the gluteus maximus. Fasciotomy of the gluteus medius and minimus is also indicated.

In the *thigh,* decompression is performed by making a longitudinal posterolateral incision and opening the fascia lata much as in the standard approach to the femur, but somewhat more posteriorly. The flexor compartment is opened below the intermuscular septum. During explorations of medial neurovascular structures, the flexor and extensor muscles may be decompressed through the same incision (Fig. 13).

In the *lower leg,* a four-compartment decompression can be performed using any of three methods:

1. Double-incision fasciotomy.
2. Parafibular decompression.
3. Fibulectomy.

The *double-incision fasciotomy* is essentially a prophylactic procedure (Mubarak, Owen 1977; Echtermeyer et al. 1980). The anterior and lateral compartments are approached through an anterolateral skin incision made in the middle part of the lower leg 2 cm anterior to the fibula. The skin is undermined somewhat proximally and distally so that the fascia can be better visualized. First the fasciae of both compartments are incised transversely in order to identify the anterior intermuscular septum. The superficial peroneal nerve is located in the lateral compartment, adjacent to the septum. To decompress both compartments, the blades of a long, blunt-pointed scissors are advanced proximally and

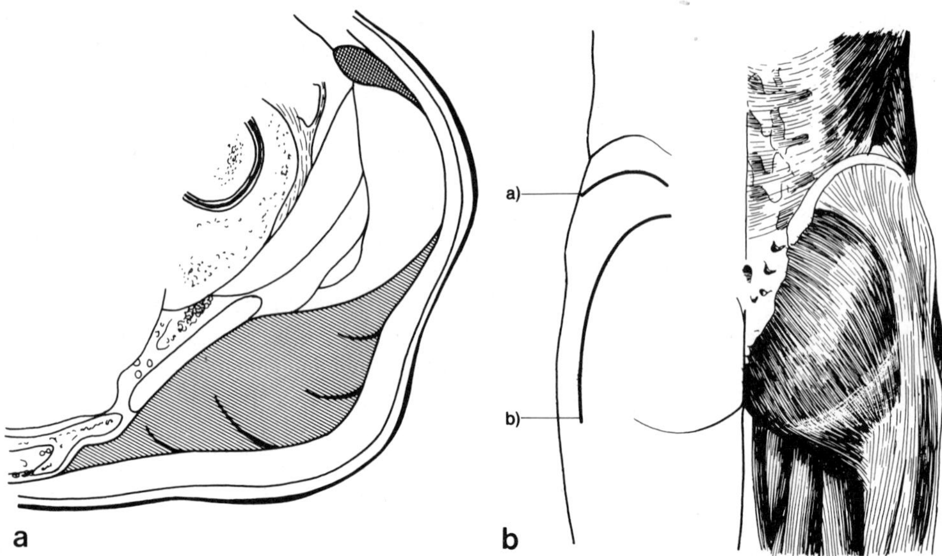

Fig. 12a, b. Compartment of the gluteal region. **a** Transverse section through the gluteal region showing the compartments of tensor fasciae latae (*darkly shaded*), gluteus medius and minimus (*unshaded*) and gluteus maximus (*lightly shaded*). **b** Skin incision for decompressing the gluteal muscles: (*a*) distal and parallel to the iliac crest, (*b*) posterior approach to the hip joint after Marcy-Fletcher-Müller

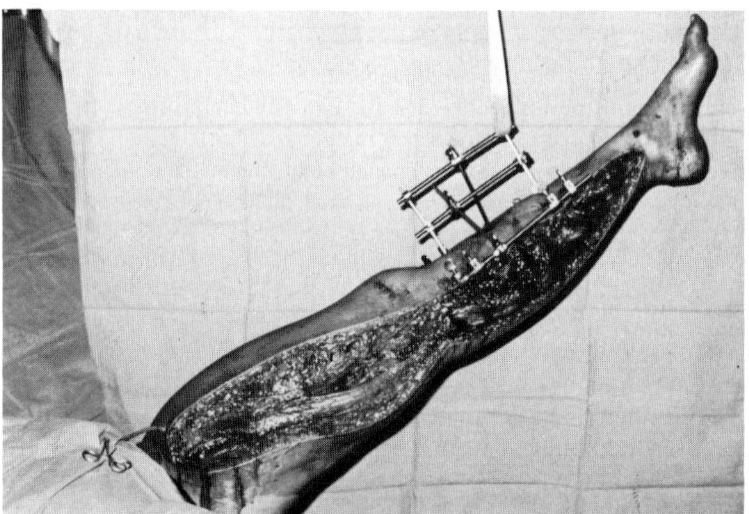

Fig. 13. Extensive compartment syndrome of the leg secondary to femoral artery rupture in a multiply injured patient. The compartments were decompressed through a medial incision of the thigh which was extended distally (atypical). The tibial fracture was stabilized with an external frame

distally. Division of the transverse crural ligament may require a second incision in some instances. The lateral compartment fasciotomy is made at the level of the fibular shaft.

The superficial and deep posterior compartments are approached through a single posteromedial skin incision in the distal part of the leg 2 cm posterior to the palpable posterior border of the tibia (Fig. 14a–c). The great saphenous vein and saphenous nerve are retracted anteriorly. A transverse incision is made in the fascia, through which the septum between the deep and superficial posterior compartments is identified. The superficial compartment is the first to be decompressed. Attention is then turned to the deep posterior compartment, whose fascia is too-often ignored. A neglected compartment syndrome in this area can result in serious functional disability. The soft-tissue coverage of the deep posterior compartment makes it inaccessible to direct palpation. However, in the distal third of the lower leg it is uncovered by the triceps surae and is readily accessible.

The *unilateral parafibular approach* enables all four compartments to be decompressed through a single skin incision (Fig. 15) (Matsen et al. 1980). The incision runs the full length of the fibula, and the lateral compartment is the first to be opened (Fig. 15a). The anterior compartment is reached by retracting the anterior skin (Fig. 15b). Retraction of the posterior skin exposes the superficial posterior compartment (Fig. 15c). After separating the lateral compartment from its posterior fascia, the peroneal muscles are retracted anteriorly and the triceps surae muscle is retracted posteriorly, placing tension on the fascia between the fibula and the deep layer of the crural fascia. It is incised to decompress the deep posterior compartment (Fig. 15d).

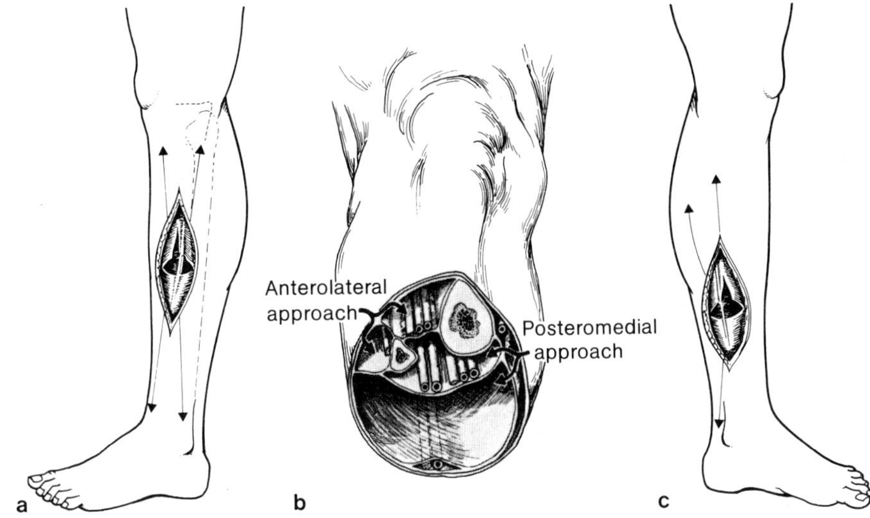

Fig. 14a–c. Double-incision prophylactic fasciotomy of the four compartments of the lower leg. **a** The lateral and anterior compartments are decompresssed through a single anterolateral skin incision. **b** Transverse section through the proximal third of the lower leg showing the anteriolateral and posteromedial approaches in schematic form. **c** The superficial and deep posterior compartments are approached through a common posteromedial skin incision

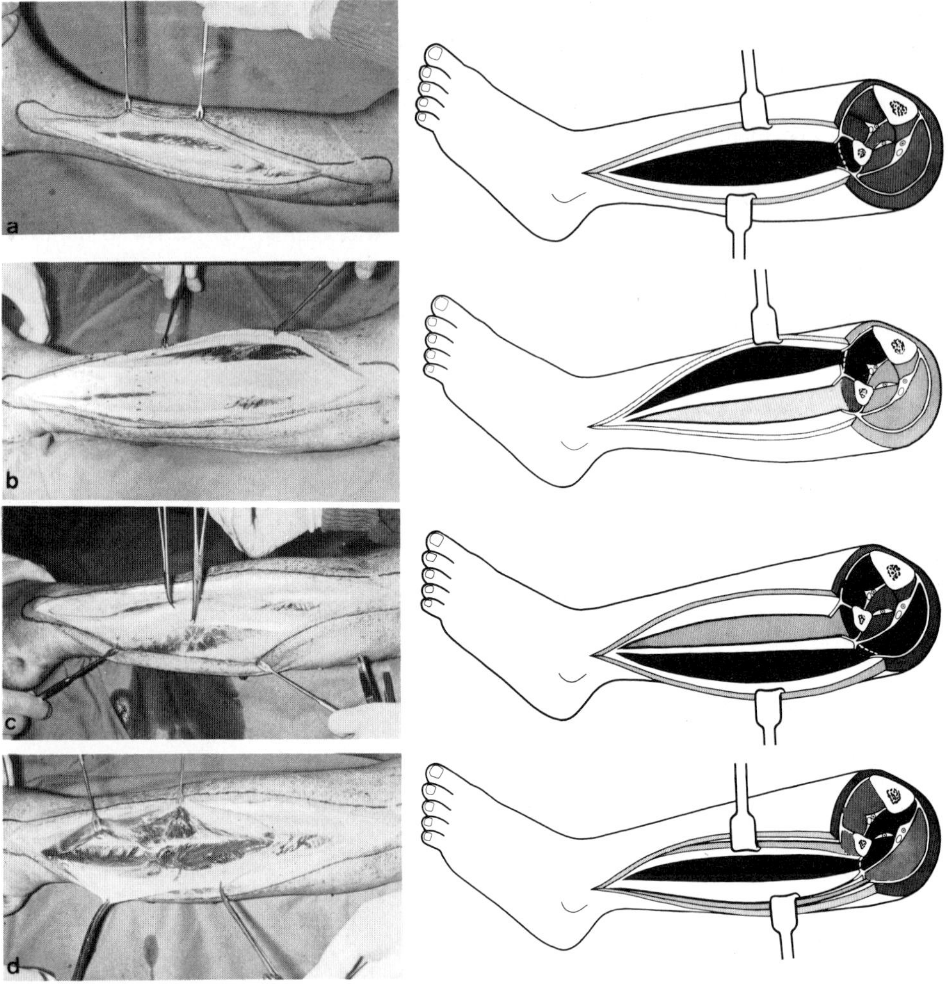

Fig. 15a–d. Four-compartment parafibular decompression after Matsen (1980). **a** The lateral compartment is opened at the level of the skin incision. **b** The anterior compartment is reached by retracting the anterior skin. **c** The superficial posterior compartment is opened by retracting the posterior skin. **d** The deep posterior compartment is reached by retracting the peroneal muscles anteriorly and the triceps surae muscle posteriorly

The more distal the location of the injury, the more important it is to divide the transverse crural ligament, as well as the cruciform ligament when performing a therapeutic fasciotomy. Compartmental ischemias of the foot also require division of these structures.

The *unilateral parafibular dermatofasciotomy* is the surest technique for effecting decompression in the face of severe soft tissue injury. Because the skin incision is more distant from the tibia than in the double-incision technique, for example, the risk of osseous infection is reduced. Exposure of the distal third of the fibula is presumed to carry a lower risk of infection than exposure of the tibia. The parafibular decompression is also less destabilizing than a bilateral incision. In addition, secondary closure is easier to procure when a unilateral incision is used. With the unilateral parafibular dermatofasciotomy, the entire surface of the wound bed is covered by muscle. A modified approach may be needed when there has been extensive degloving of the extremity. In this case a straight midline incision is made through the contused area so that skin nutrition will not be further disrupted by the destruction of perforating blood vessels. A four-compartment decompression is than effected through a double-incision fasciotomy.

A *fibulectomy* (Fig. 16) allows all four compartments to be opened through a single incision (Kelly, Whitesides 1967; Ernst, Kaufer 1971; Feagin, White 1973). The fibular resection is subperiostal and extends from a point 8 cm above the lateral malleolus to just

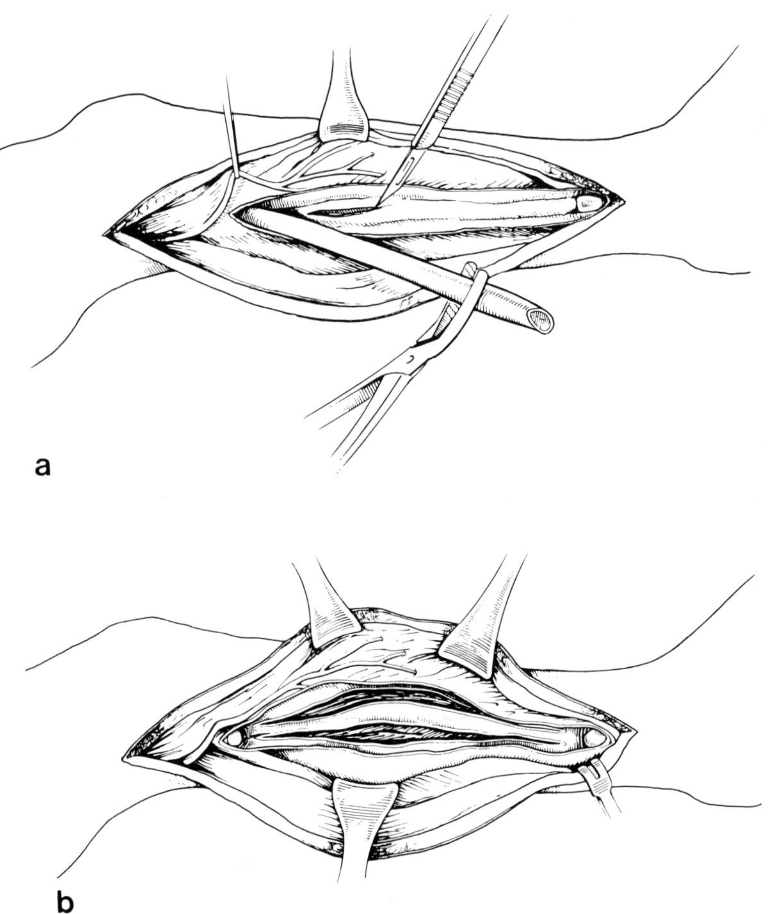

Fig. 16a, b. Fibulectomy as a means of decompressing the four compartments of the lower leg. **a** Subtotal resection of the fibula. **b** Condition following fibulectomy and opening of all four compartments

below the proximal tibiofibular syndesmosis. However, we feel that the extent of the surgery and the relatively high risk of peroneal nerve injury make this technique inferior to parafibular decompression. Loss of stability is another disadvantage of the fibulectomy.

In the *foot* (Fig. 17), decompression requires not only that the compartments of the short pedal muscles be opened, but also that the skin be adequately released. The structure of the plantar region causes blood and lymph pooling to occur mainly in the dorsal area of the foot (Lanz, von Wachsmuth 1972). Decompression of the skin and muscles is indicated for all serious foot injuries, with or without osseous involvement. The lateral approach, which includes division of the lower extensor retinaculum, passes between the 4th and 5th rays over the dorsum of the foot. The skin over the 1st metatarsal bone is also incised if necessary.

The three compartments in the plantar region of the foot are decompressed by dividing the plantar aponeurosis transversely near its origin on the calcaneus.

11. Results

We have reviewed 123 compartment syndromes, including late referrals, which we treated from 1978 to 1982 (Oestern, Echtermeyer 1982). Ninty-six of these involved the lower leg, 11 the thigh, 8 the upper arm, and 5 the forearm. One compartment syndrome involved the gluteal region (Table 1). The age distribution of the patients showed a definite peak between the ages of 20 and 30 years (Fig. 18). A fasciotomy was performed in 95 patients, and 8 patients were treated conservatively (Table 2). Late sequelae developed in 36 patients, 35 of whom had a compartment syndrome of the lower leg. Twenty-nine displayed

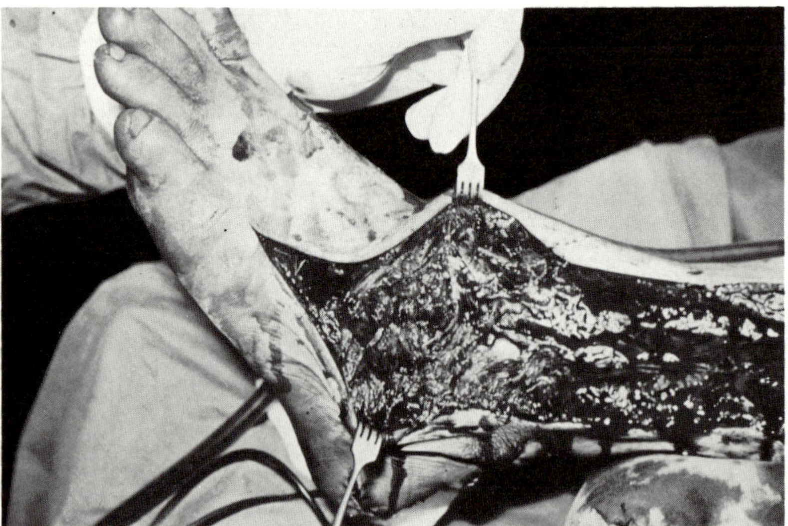

Fig. 17. Release of the skin and subcutaneous tissue in frank compartment syndrome of the foot following a severe crush injury with tarsal and metatarsal fractures

Table 1. Compartment syndromes (n = 123); 1978–1982

Lower leg	96
Thigh	11
Upper arm	8
Forearm	5
Gluteal region	1
Hand	1
Foot	1

weak dorsiflexion of the foot, four had a claw-toe deformity, and nine complained of sensory losses (Table 3).

Analyzing the sequelae that occurred after fasciotomy, we find that late changes, developed in only three patients who underwent a fasciotomy within the first six hours after their injury. By contrast, late changes occurred in 22 patients in whom decompression was

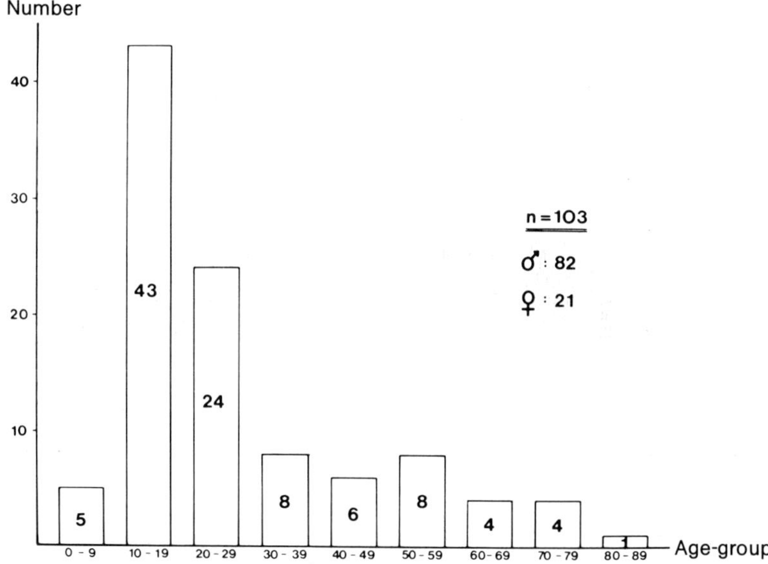

Fig. 18. Distribution of 103 compartment syndromes by age group

Table 2. Timing of fasciotomy in 95 patients with compartment syndromes (n = 95)

< 6 h	39
6 – 12 h	8
12 – 24 h	23
> 24 h	25

Table 3. Late sequelae of compartment syndromes

Weak dorsiflexion of the foot	n = 20
Weak dorsiflexion of the big toe	n = 6
Sensory losses	n = 9
Flexion contracture	n = 4

delayed beyond 24 hours (Table 4). Ten patients eventually had to undergo an amputation; in none of these cases had a decompressive fasciotomy been performed within the first six hours (1 within the first 12 hours, 2 between 12 and 24 hours, and 7 more than 24 hours postinjury).

Eight patients were treated nonoperatively. Seven developed late sequelae, and only one recovered completely.

Thirteen patients developed an infection. In 11 of these the fasciotomy had been performed more than 12 hours postinjury (Table 5).

Table 4. Distribution of late sequelae as a function of the timing of surgical decompression

< 6 h	3
6 – 12 h	4
12 – 24 h	7
> 24 h	22

Table 5. Infection rates as a function of the timing of fasciotomy in 95 operatively-treated compartment syndromes

< 6 h	0
6 – 12 h	2
> 12 h	11

12. Conclusions

Although the disastrous consequences of a neglected compartment syndrome have been known since the time of Volkmann (1881), the importance of the syndrome as a disease entity or trauma complication is still not fully appreciated.

Reports vary as to the prevalence of compartment syndromes in the lower leg, which is the area of predilection for this condition. In a series of 905 tibial fractures, Heim and Grete (1972) observed only 7 compartment syndromes (0.8%). Ellis (1958) reported an incidence of 2.5%. Owen and Tsimboukis (1967) found the syndrome in 10%. Our own investigations indicate that the condition develops in 17% of all tibial fractures. The discrepancies result from differences in the mechanisms of the trauma. In the Heim study (1972), for example, almost all patients in the series had suffered skiing accidents, whereas in our studies, vehicular accidents with major soft tissue trauma (e.g., bumper injuries) accounted for the great majority of tibial fractures.

Decompressive fasciotomy is an emergency procedure, and facilities for this operation should be available at all times. Promptness has a critical bearing on the prognosis. According to McQuillen and Nolan (1968) and Matsen and Clawson (1975), disturbances of muscular microcirculation that persist longer than 12 hours produce significant motor and sensory deficits as well as myogenic contractures. Keays (1981) states that, based on his experience, good results are obtained only if decompression is performed within 6 hours of the onset of a compartment syndrome. He further states that permanent defects may be expected after 8 hours, and that amputation will very likely be needed if surgery is delayed beyond 12 hours. Of his ten patients treated by fibulectomy, only four had a good end result.

Most findings on the temporal relationship between circulatory impairment and reparative tissue tolerance are based on experimental total ischemia. Nerves showed functional deficits after only 30 minutes' ischemia. Irreversible pareses developed after 12–24 hours of complete ischemia (Holmes et al. 1944; Malan 1963). Compensatable, partial myogenic disturbances were observed after only 2–4 hours' ischemia, and an irreversible loss of function after 4–12 hours (Harman 1948; Whitesides 1971). These findings are consistent with our own clinical observation that permanent functional deficits arise within 4–6 hours of the onset of a frank, untreated compartment syndrome.

The logical conclusion from a therapeutic standpoint is to normalize the blood flow by lowering the intracompartmental pressure. Except for the tibial region, the incisions recommended for surgical decompression will also provide sufficient accesss for internal fixation of the fractured bone.

The greater the problems of soft-tissue management would be with a nonoperative approach, the stronger the indication for operative fixation. Because the standard approaches for decompressing the lower leg are not easily reconciled with the incisions for internal stabilization, external fixation offers a valuable alternative in the tibial region.

The excision of necrotic muscle is especially important for the prevention of infection, which all too often necessitates amputation of the extremity (Hicks 1964; Nicoll 1964). It is also an effective means of preventing the adherent cicatrization and consequent contracture of muscle tissue that is still intact at operation (Ramadier 1981).

Late sequelae from compartment syndromes are still alarmingly common and are due largely to the delayed recognition of these syndromes, whose general management was described as early as 1911 by Bardenheuer in a lengthy monograph.

References

1. Akeson WH, Hargens AR, Garfin SR, Mubarak SJ (1981) Muscle compartment syndromes and snake bites. In: Hargens AR (ed) Tissue fluid pressure and composition. Williams and Wilkins, Baltimore, p 215
2. Aston H (1975) The effect of increased tissue pressure on blood flow. Clin Orthop Relat Res 113:15
3. Bardenheuer B (1911) Die Entstehung und Behandlung der ischaemischen Muskelkontur und Gangrän. Dtsch Z Chir 108:44
4. Benjamin A (1957) The relief of traumatic arterial spasm in threatened Volkmann's ischemic contracture. J Bone Joint Surg 39B:711

5. Buck-Gramcko D (1974) Ischämische Kontrakturen am Unterarm und Hand. Handchir 6:141
6. Burton AC (1951) On the physical equilibrium of small blood vessels. Physiol Rev 34: 619
7. Eaton RG, Green WT (1972) Epimysiotomy and fasciotomy in the treatment of Volkmann's ischemic contracture. Orthop Clin North Am 3:175
8. Echtermeyer V, Godt P, Muhr G (1980) Das posttraumatische Muskelkompressionssyndrom. Pathophysiologie und Technik der Dekompression. Hefte Unfallheilkd 148: 192
9. Echtermeyer V, Muhr G, Oestern HJ, Tscherne H (1982) Chirurgische Behandlung des Kompartment-Syndroms. Unfallheilkd 85:114
10. Ellis H (1958) Disabilities after tibial shaft fractures. J Bone Joint Surg 40B:190
11. Ernst CB, Kaufer H (1971) Fibulectomy – Fasciotomy. J Trauma 11:365
12. Feagin JA, White AA (1973) Volkmanns ischemia treated by transfibular fasciotomy. Milit Med 138:497
13. Feigl EO (1974) Physics of the cardiovascular system. In: Ruch TC, Patton HD (ed) Physiology and Biophysics. Circulation, Respiration and Fluid Balance, Vol 2. Saunders, Philadelphia London Toronto
14. Finochietto R (1920) Retraccion des Volkmann de los musculos intrinsecos de la mano. Bol Trab Soc Chir (Buenos Aires) 4:31
15. Foisie PS (1942) Volkmann's ischemic conctracture. An analysis of its proximate mechanism. N Engl J Med 226:671
16. Fuhrmann FA, Crismon JM (1951) Early changes in distribution of sodium potassium and water in rabbit muscles following release of tourniquets. Am J Physiol 166:424
17. Gardner RC (1970) Inpending Volkmann's contracture following minor trauma to the palm of the hand. A theory of pathogenesis. Clin Orthop Relat Res 72:261
18. Garfin SR, Mubarak SJ, Evans KL, Hargens AR, Akeson WH (1981) Quantification of intracompartmental pressure and volume under plastercasts. J Bone Joint Surg 63A: 449
19. Garfin SR, Tipton CM, Mubarak SJ, Woo SLY, Hargens AR, Akeson WH (1981) The role of fascia in the maintenance of muscle tension and pressure. A Appl Physiol (in press)
20. Gaspard DJ, Kohl RD (1975) Compartmental syndromes in which the skin is limiting boundary. Clin Orthop 113:65
21. Goodfellow J, Fearn CRDA, Mathens JM (1978) Decompression of forearm compartment syndromes. Clin Orthop 134:225
22. Hargens AR, Akeson HW, Mubarak SJ et al. (1978) Fluid balance within the canine anterolateral compartment and its relationship to compartment syndromes. J Bone Joint Surg 60A:499
23. Harman JW, Gwinn RP (1948) The recovery of skeletal muscle fibers from acute ischemia as determined by histologic and chemical methods. Am J Pathol 25:741
24. Heim U, Grete W (1972) Das Tibialis-anterior-Syndrom nach Osteosynthese am Unterschenkel. Helv Chir Acta 39:667
25. Hicks JH (1964) Amputation in fractures of the tibia. J Bone Joint Surg 46B:388
26. Holden CEA (1975) Compartmental syndromes following trauma. Clin Orthop 113:95
27. Holmes W, Highet WB, Seddon JH (1944) Ischaemic nerve lesions occuring in Volkmann's contracture. Br J Surg 32:259
28. Keays AC (1981) Fibulectomy – Fasciotomy. J Bone Joint Surg 63B:478
29. Kelly RP, Whitesides TE Jr (1967) Transfibular route for fasciotomy of the leg. J Bone Joint Surg 49A:1022
30. Kjellmer J (1964) An indirect method for estimating tissue pressure with special reference to tissue pressure in muscle during exercise. Acta Plupiol Scand 62:31
31. Lanz J, v. Wachsmuth W (1972) Praktische Anatomie. Bein und Statik. Springer, Berlin Heidelberg New York
32. Lanz M (1979) Ischämische Muskelnekrosen. Hefte Unfallheilkd 139

33. Malan E, Tattom G (1963) Physio- and anatomo-pathology of acute ischemia of the extremities. J Cardiovasc Surg 17:212
34. Matsen FA III, Clawson DK (1975) The deep posterior compartmental syndrome of the leg. J Bone Joint Surg 57A:34
35. Matsen FA, Mayo KA, Sheridan GW, Krugmire RB (1976) Monitoring of transmuscular pressure. Surgery 79:702
36. Matsen FA III (1980) Compartmental syndromes. Grune & Stratton, New York London Toronto Sydney San Francisco
37. Matsen FA III, Winquist RA, Krugmire RB Jr (1980) Diagnosis and management of compartmental syndromes. J Bone Joint Surg 62A:286
38. Matsen FA III, Wyss CR, Krugmire RB et al. (1980) The effects of limb elevation and dependency on local arteriovenous gradients in normal human limbs with particular reference to limbs with increased tissue pressure. Clin Orthop Relat Res 150:187
39. May H (1970) Ischämische Kontrakturen der unteren Extremität bei Kindern und Erwachsenen. Hefte Unfallheilkd 102:142
40. McQuillan WM, Nolan B (1968) Ischaemia complicating injury. J Bone Joint Surg 50B:482
41. Meier F, Heinz C (1974) Tibialis-anterior Syndrom nach Frakturen am Unterschenkel. Chir Praxis 18:297
42. Mubarak SJ, Owen CA (1977) Double-incision fasciotomy of the leg for decompression in compartment-syndromes. J Bone Joint Surg 59A:184
43. Mubarak SJ, Owen CA, Hargens AR, Garetto LP, Akeson WH (1978) Acute compartment syndromes: Diagnosis and treatment with the aid of wick catheter. J Bone Joint Surg 60A:1091
44. Mubarak SJ, Hargens AR, Lee YF, Lundblad AK, Castle GSP, Rorabeck CH (1981) Slit catheter – a new technique for measuring tissue fluid pressure and quantifying muscle contraction. 27th Annual Meeting, Orthopedic Res Soc, Las Vegas, NV
45. Mubarak SJ, Hargens AR (1981) Compartment-Syndromes and Volkmann's Contracture. Saunders. Philadelphia London Toronto
46. Mummenthaler M, Mummenthaler A, Medici V (1969) Das Tibialis-anterior-Syndrom nach Operationen am Unterschenkel. Seine Fehldiagnose als Peroneusparese. Arch Orthop Unfall-Chir 66:201
47. Nicoll EA (1965) Fractures of the tibial shaft. J Bone Joint Surg 46B:373
48. Oestern HJ, Echtermeyer V (1982) Behandlung des Kompartmentsyndroms und Ergebnisse. Langenbecks Arch Chir 358
49. Owen R, Tsimboukis B (1967) Ischaemia complicating closed tibial and fibula shaft fractures. J Bone Joint Surg 49B:268
50. Owen CA, Mubarak SJ, Hargens AR, Ratherford L, Garetto LP, Akeson WH (1978) Intramuscular pressure with limb compression. Clarification of the pathogenesis of the drug-induced compartment-syndrome/crush syndrome. N Engl J Med 300:1169
51. Pernkopf E (1980) Atlas der topographischen und angewandten Anatomie des Menschen: Brust, Bauch und Extremitäten. Urban und Schwarzenberg, München Wien Baltimore
52. Ramadier IO (1981) Syndrome ischemique post-traumatique des loges de la jambe. Int Orthop 5:91
53. Reneman RS (1975) The anterior and the lateral compartmental syndrome of the leg due to intensiv use of muscles. Clin Orthop 113:69
54. Ryder HW, Molle WE, Ferris EB (1953) The influence of the collapsibility of veins on venous pressure, including a new procedure for measuring tissue pressure. J Clin Invest 23:334
55. Tscherne H (1982) Editorial Unfallheilkunde 85
56. Volkmann R (1881) Die ischämischen Muskellähmungen und -kontrakturen. Zentralbl Chir 8:801
57. Waiber P, Nigst H, Hess (1960) Spätzustand nach akutem traumatischen Tibialis-anterior-Syndrom. Schweiz Med Wochenschr 90:700

58. Wells J, Templeton J (1977) Femoral neuropathy associated with anticoagulant therapy. Clin Orthop 124:155
59. Whitesides TE, Hirada H, Morimoto K (1971) The response of skeletal muscle to temporary ischemia: an experimental study. J Bone Joint Surg 53A:1027
60. Whitesides TE Jr, Honey TC, Morimoto K, Hirada H (1975) Tissue pressure measurements as a determinant for the need of fasciotomy. Clin Orthop 113:43
61. Whitesides TE, Hirada H, Morimoto K (1977) Compartment syndromes and the role of fasciotomy, its parameters and techniques. Instructional Course Lectures. The American Academy of Orthopedic Surgeons Vol 26. Mosby, St Louis
62. Wissing H (1980) Die Bedeutung der Compartmentdruckmessung in der Beurteilung des Weichteilschadens am Unterschenkel. Hefte Unfallheilkd 148:499
63. Wissing H, Schmit-Neuerburg KP (1982) Diagnose und Differentialdiagnose des Kompartment-Syndroms. Unfallheilkd 85:133
64. Zweifach SS, Hargens AR, Evans KI, Gonsalves MR, Smith RK, Mubarak SJ, Akeson WM (1980) Skeletal muscle necrosis in pressurized compartments associated with hemorrhagic hypotension. J Trauma 20:941

External Articular Transfixation for Joint Injuries with Severe Soft Tissue Damage

D. Rogge

1. Introduction

The severity of an extremity injury is determined to a large extent by the degree of concomitant soft tissue damage especially when it occurs near the joints. Sound therapeutic planning is only possible, if the extent of both open and closed soft tissue injuries are fully evaluated (Tscherne and Brüggemann 1976). The choice of treatment is decisively influenced by the nature, localization, and severity of concomitant soft tissue trauma.

With all extensive injuries, special immobilization is required in order to promote healing and accelerate functional recovery.

Therapeutic Goals

The following requirements for this type of injury are mandatory and often difficult to fulfill:

a) Secure immobilization
b) Adequate positioning
c) Good accessibility
d) Continuous observation
e) Optimal hygiene.

With ordinary conservative methods of splinting and plaster immobilization, it is very difficult to satisfy all these goals to the desired degree. External fixation is ideally suited to provide stable immobilization while allowing unrestricted access to the injured area.

The principle of treatment is temporary external transfixation of the injured joint (Rogge et al. 1980; Schmelzeisen et al. 1982).

This mode of fixation can be applied to any of the major joints, though it is most commonly used on the knee and ankle joints. It has additional prophylactic value in the prevention of the equinus deformity of the ankle.

2. Indications and Principles of Treatment

Along with the known principles of intraarticular fracture management and the treatment of severe soft tissue injuries, special problems related to indications and management are connected with the following types of articular and periarticular injury:

a) Fractures with severe soft tissue damage that are amenable to stable internal fixation.
b) Fractures with severe soft tissue damage that cannot be stabilized by internal fixation alone, especially when bone loss has occured.

c) Fractures in which the extent and localization of soft tissue damage or the fracture itself prohibit internal fixation.
d) Joint disruptions with severe soft tissue injury.

Remarks on a): With fractures allowing stable internal fixation, external transfixation is done solely for the treatment of soft tissue lesions. The external fixator can be applied in either a full-frame or half-frame configuration, and may be removed after soft tissues have healed (Fig. 1).

Remarks on b): Fractures with large comminuted zones or bone loss in proximity to a joint occasionally cannot be adequately stabilized by internal fixation alone. Buttressing or

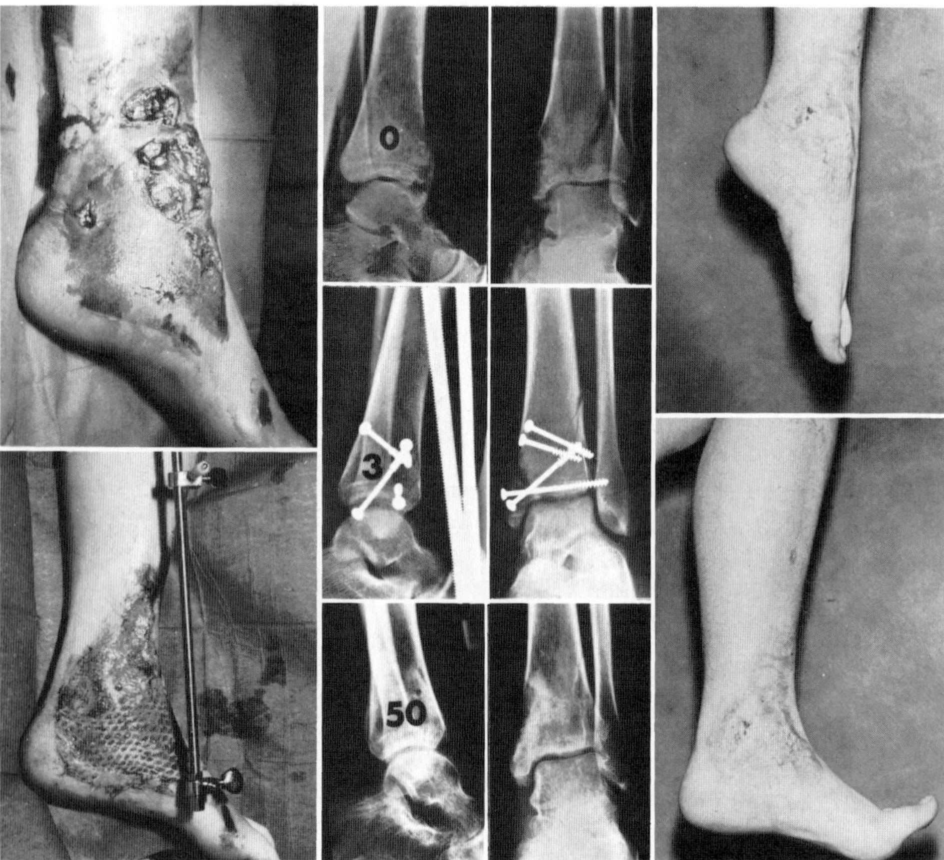

Fig. 1. Soft tissue stabilization with external transfixation: Severe soft tissue injuries and burns associated with a distal intraarticular fracture of the tibia. The fracture was fixed with compression screws, soft tissues stabilized for 4 weeks with a simple transfixing bilateral frame. Mesh graft was used for wound closure. Functional result at 50 weeks was excellent

bridging plates cannot always be securely attached close to a joint and, especially near the knee joint, very large levering forces exist.

In these cases external articular transfixation is valuable not only in immobilizing the soft tissues but also in giving added stability to the fracture. The main periarticular fragment, which cannot be adequately stabilized with internal fixation, is effectually lengthened and stabilized beyond the joint area by the external fixator (Fig. 2).

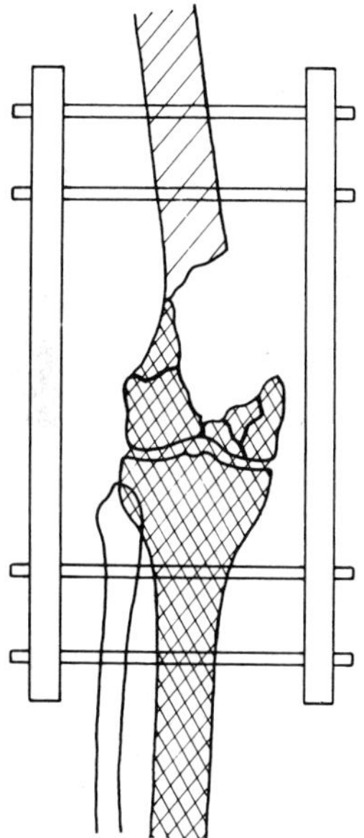

Fig. 2. Fracture stabilization with external transfixation (*schematic*): Periarticular fragments that cannot be stabilized with internal fixation are effectually lengthened beyong the immobilized joint and stabilized by the transfixing frame

The best stability is achieved by applying the fixator in a three-dimensional or triangular configuration (Fig. 3). Often a simple half frame applied to the anterior aspect of the limb can provide adequate stability (Fig. 4). The fixator is removed only when fracture healing has progressed to the point where osseous stability is satisfactory.

Remarks on c): Fractures which are only treatable by external fixation due to the extent and location of soft tissue trauma may be stabilized by either of the two methods mentioned above.

If articular transfixation is not needed to stabilize the fracture, it is nevertheless of value in promoting soft tissue healing. In these cases a simple configuration may be used, preferably one whose transarticular element can be easily removed following soft tissue healing without disturbing the fracture-stabilizing components (Fig. 5).

If articular transfixation is required to stabilize the fracture, the frame which usually is three-dimensional is extended beyond the joint. The design of the frame should allow removal of the transarticular element when fracture healing progresses.

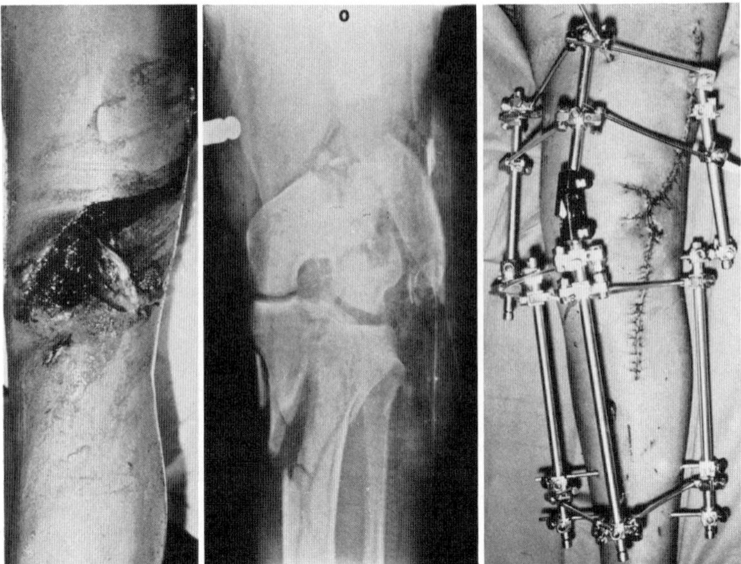

Fig. 3. Fracture stabilization with external transfixation: Grade III open comminuted fracture of the distal femur with bone loss and ipsilateral comminuted fracture of the proximal tibia with severe closed soft tissue injury. Following primary soft tissue debridement and minimal internal fixation, the fracture was stabilized externally by means of a triangular frame with removable transarticular component

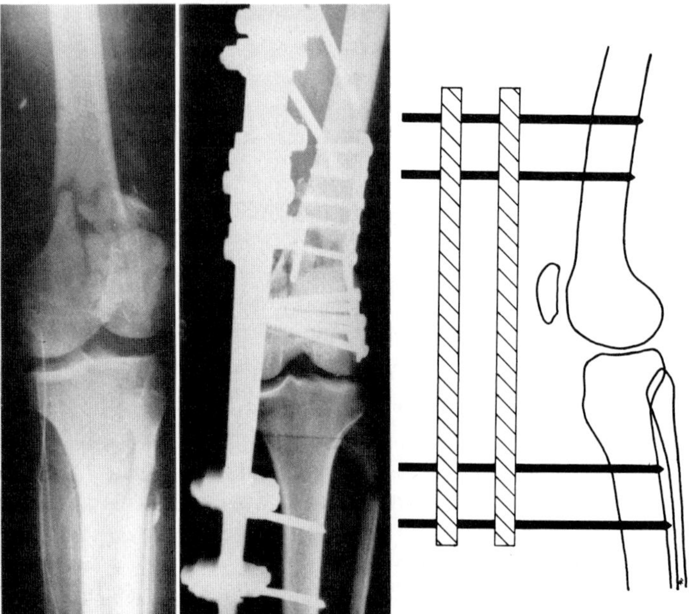

Fig. 4. Transfixation by anterior unilateral half frame: Grade III open comminuted distal femoral fracture with bone loss associated with severe closed soft tissue trauma in the lower leg. The fracture was fixed internally with a condylar buttress plate and then stabilized externally by applying a double-rod half frame anteriorly across the joint

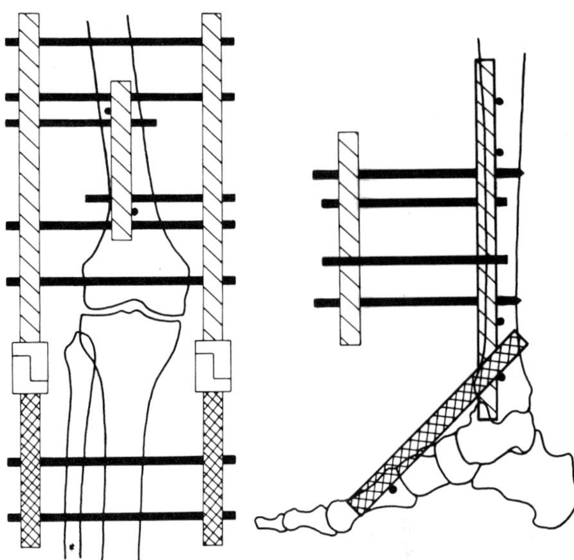

Fig. 5. External transfixation used to supplement the external fixation of a fracture (*schematic*): Removal of the joint-bridging component of the fixator (*cross-hatched*) is possible without affecting the remaining frame

Remarks on d): In dislocations and joint disruptions with severe soft tissue injury, external articular transfixation serves as an ideal principle. It immobilizes the sutured capsular and ligamentous structures, provides stability for healing tissues, and protects repairs that have been made on injured nerves and blood vessels.

Once the dislocation has been reduced, highest priority is given to injuries of the major blood vessels. Revascularization of the injured extremity is the major concern. Specific management will vary, but in most cases the correct procedure is to apply the external fixator only after vascular repairs have been completed. However, in exceptional cases where instability is extreme, it may be advisable to apply the external transfixation before repairing the vessels. A quickly-applied external fixator will maintain the reduction and facilitate vascular repairs.

The duration of ischemia can be significantly reduced by the immediate insertion of an intraluminal shunt.

Pure dislocations with severe soft tissue injury or neurovascular lesions, unaccompanied by fractures, are seen most frequently in the knee joint. Generally a bilateral frame or anterior half frame gives sufficient immobilization, although a triangular frame may be necessary in cases of severe instability. Under no circumstance should the fixator be used to apply axial compression. Most cases require about six weeks of immobilization.

Removal of the external transfixation is always followed by a period of intensive rehabilitation of the joint. In the initial phase, main emphasis is placed upon continuous passive mobilization of the joint be a motor-driven splint.

Technique of External Articular Transfixation

The configuration of the transfixing frame should conform to the specific stability requirements of the situation without restricting access to the injured area. Since constant pressure on the articular surfaces combined with strict immobilization leads to secondary articular degeneration, the frame should not exert compression across the joint (Refior et al. 1976; Finsterbush et al. 1975).

The *wrist* is bridged with a half frame. Two half pins (Schanz screws) are each inserted into the distal radius and into the second metacarpal bone from the dorsomedial side and axially stabilized by means of a single connecting rod. To avoid injury to the extensor apparatus, the pins are inserted obliquely at an angle of 45° radial to the sagittal plane (Fig. 6).

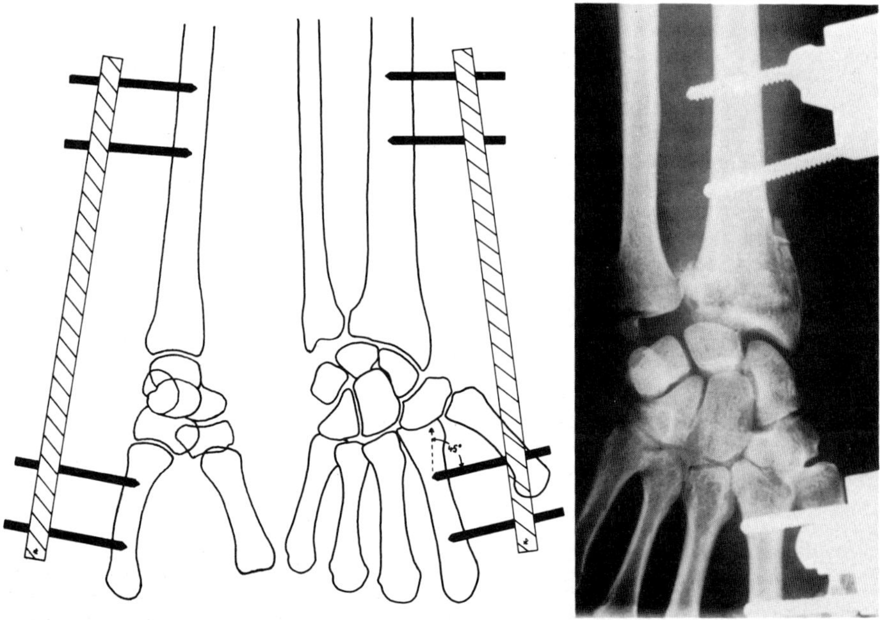

Fig. 6. Transfixation of the wrist: Anterior half frame angled 45° toward the radial side. The proximal pins are anchored in the radius, the distal pins in the second metacarpal

In the *knee joint* a bilateral frame usually is sufficient if bony conditions are stable. It is held in place by two pairs of transfixing pins (Steinmann pins) inserted proximal and distal to the joint (Fig. 7). In certain cases an anterior half frame can provide adequate immobilization (Fig. 4). Often a simple tubular connecting rod will suffice (Fig. 8). In the presence of an unstable fracture or extensive tears of knee ligaments, a triangular frame may be necessary to preserve rotational alignment (Fig. 9).

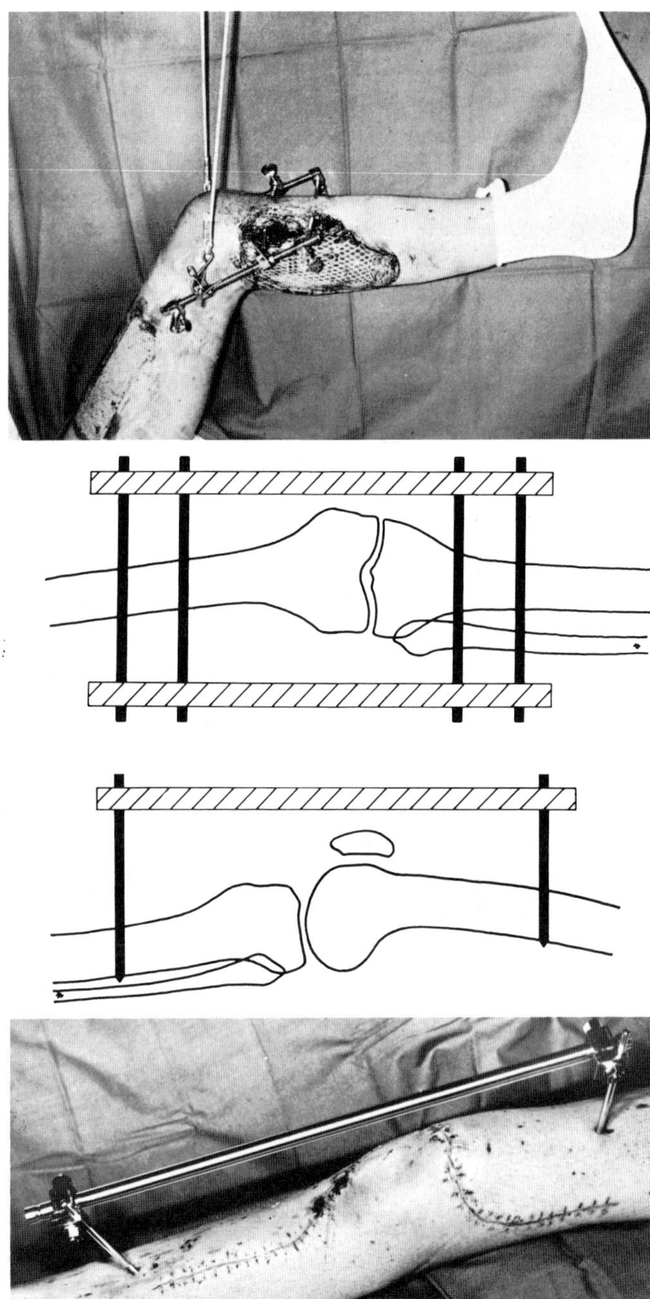

Fig. 7. Transfixation of the knee joint: Bilateral frame, applied here for a grade III open dislocation of the knee

Fig. 8. Transfixation of the knee joint: An anterior half frame is sufficient, when instability is not severe. A distal, internally-fixed grade III open comminuted femoral fracture with damage to the extensor apparatus has been stabilized. The connecting rod may be removed to permit therapeutic exercise

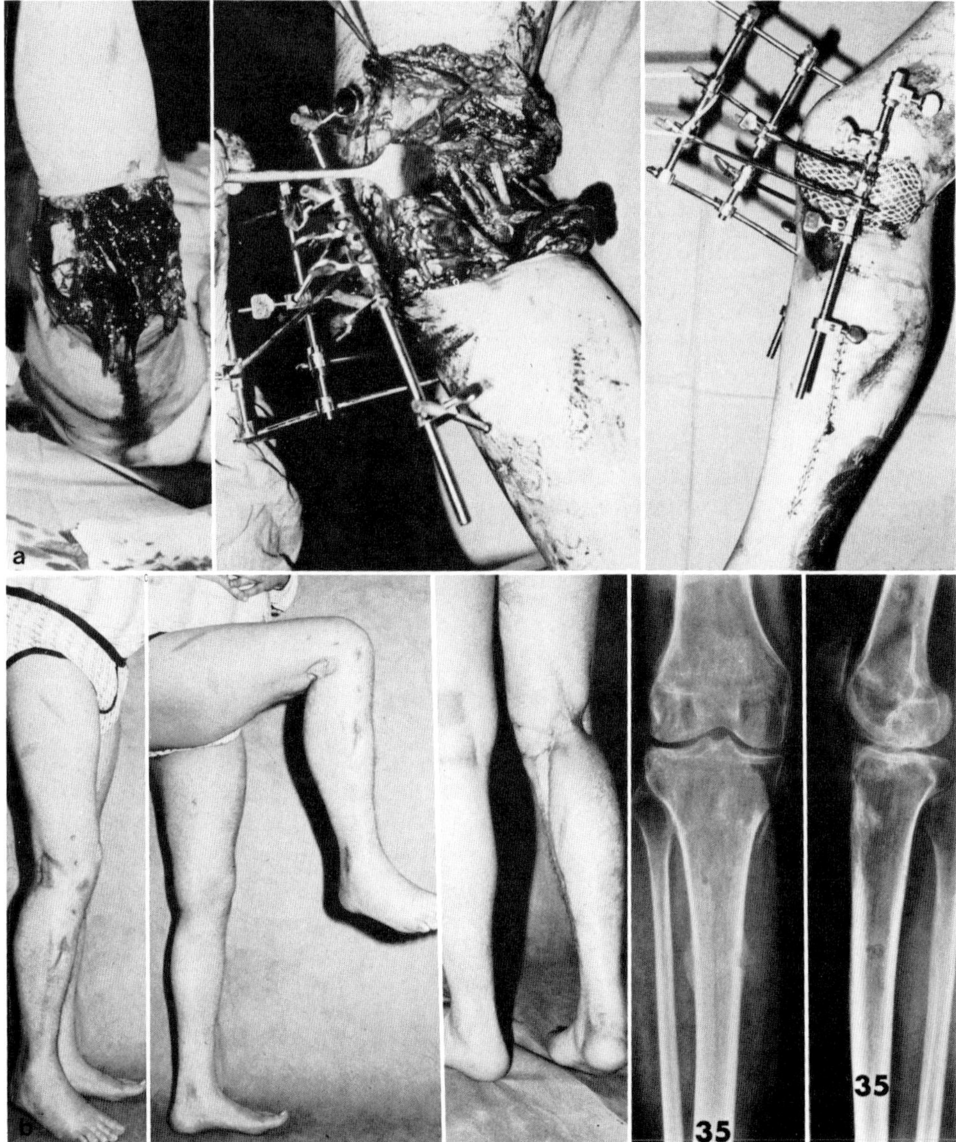

Fig. 9a, b. Transfixation of the knee joint: Three-dimensional frame, applied here for a massive grade III open posterior knee disruption with tears of the popliteal artery and vein. The vessels were repaired by end-to-end anastomosis, a fasciotomy was performed, and meshed split-thickness skin graft was applied secondarily. Function after 35 weeks was good

For anatomical reasons, transfixation of the *ankle joint* and *tarsus* generally can be accomplished with a simple bilateral frame and two transfixing pins. Depending on the type of injury present, it may be most advantageous to insert the distal pin extraarticular through the base or heads of metatarsals I–IV, through the distal tarsal bones, or through the neck of the talus (Fig. 10). Any of these placements may be used without significant consequences.

A more stable configuration for ankle injuries, especially when an intraarticular fracture is present, is a V-shaped frame incorporating two extra rods and an additional transfixing pin through the calcaneus. Besides enhancing stability, this arrangement produces a slight distraction of the calcaneus which relieves pressure from the ankle joint when the foot is raised against gravity or against an existing equinus deformity (Fig. 10 and 11).

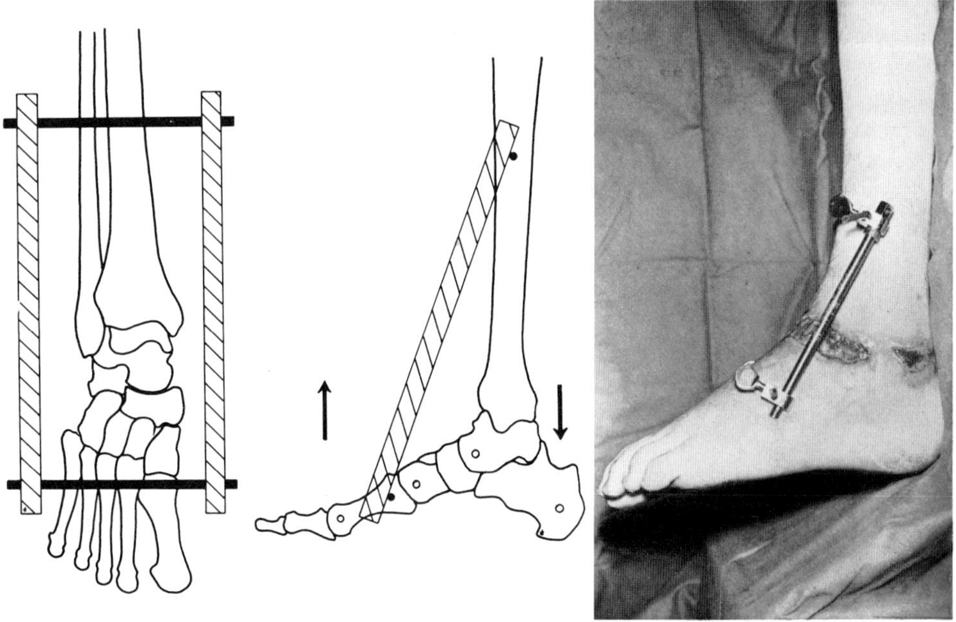

Fig. 10. Transfixation of the ankle joint: Simple bilateral frame. The distal transfixing pin may be inserted through the head or bases of the metatarsals, through the distal row of tarsal bones, or through the neck of the talus, as desired. Pressure can be taken off from the ankle joint by inserting an additional pin through the calcaneus to obtain slight distraction (cf. Fig. 11)

If the nature of the fracture or soft tissue injury prohibits the placement of a Steinmann pin through the distal tibia, a special arrangement may be utilized in which the fixation frame is applied in the frontal plane, anchored distally by a transmetatarsal pin, and supported proximally by a Schanz screw inserted into the anterior distal tibia (Fig. 12).

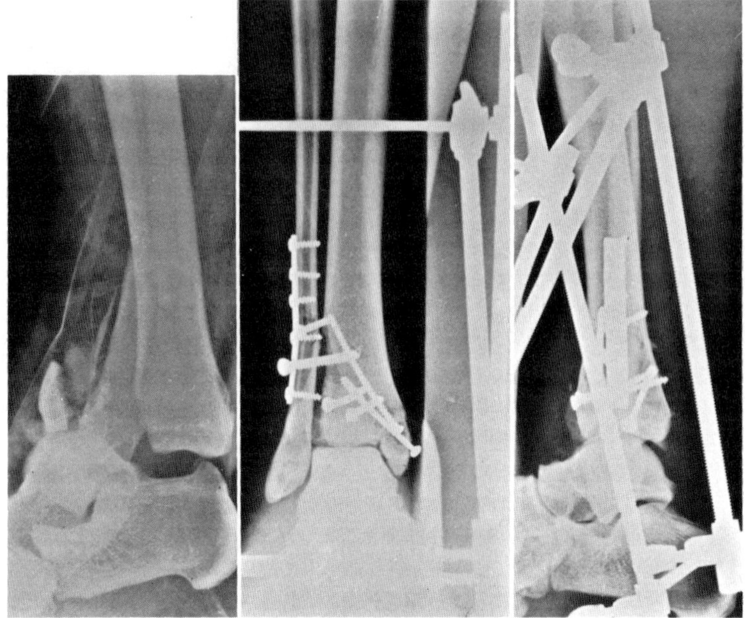

Fig. 11. Transfixation of the ankle joint for an intraarticular fracture: Distraction of the calcaneus is useful for relieving pressure on the fractured joint surface, especially in pilon fractures (cf. Fig. 10)

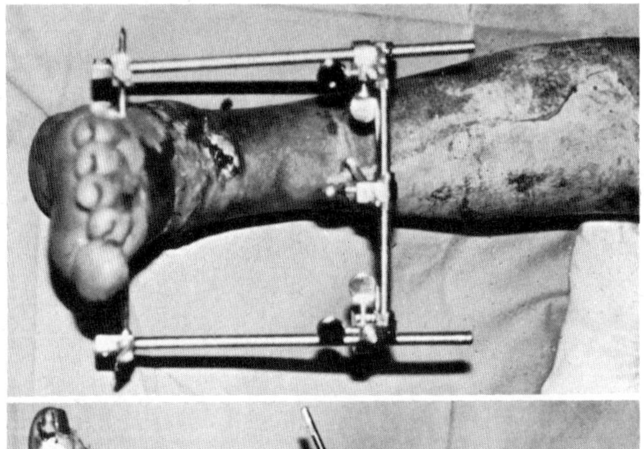

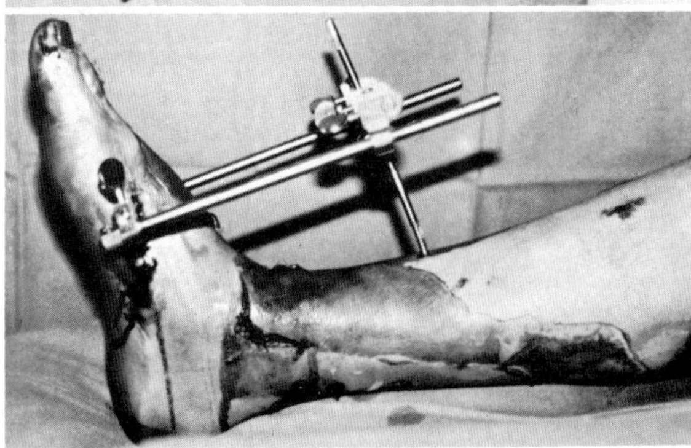

Fig. 12. Transfixation of the ankle joint with a special frame: III° burn associated with an ankle joint fracture-dislocation. This arrangement is useful if soft tissue conditions are unusually precarious and stability is reasonably good. Trauma is minimized by inserting a single Schanz screw into the distal tibia

4. Clinical Material

Fractures

From July 1974 to December 1982 external articular transfixation was applied to 81 joints in 74 patients ranging in age from 7 to 86 years. The series included 6 elbow joints, 13 wrist joints, 3 hip joints, 17 knee joints, and 42 ankle joints (Table 1).

Forty-four patients had an open grade III soft tissue injury, 8 with associated neurovascular damage. Eight patients had a closed severe soft tissue injury, 2 with neurovascular lesions and 2 with a compartment syndrome.

Eleven arterial reconstructions, 4 involving the posterior tibial artery, were required. A fasciotomy had to be performed in 19 cases. In 51 cases the skin was closed secondarily with mesh grafts, preceded in 38 cases by temporary coverage with Epigard. Plastic procedures utilizing cutaneous or musculocutaneous flaps were performed in 7 patients, one of whom required a microvascular anastomosis.

The mean duration of transfixation was 5.1 (3–8) weeks for the knee joint and 7.1 (1.5–22) weeks for the ankle joint. The longest period was 22 weeks.

Table 1. External articular transfixation for fractures. July 1974–December 1982

Elbow joint	Wrist	Hip joint	Knee	Ankle joint
6	13	3	17	42

Grade III soft tissue injury:		open:	44 patients	
		closed:	8 patients	
Vascular repairs:	11		Epigard:	38
Fasciotomy primary:	16		Secondary suture:	6
secondary:	3		Mesh graft:	51
			Flap:	7
Mean duration of transfixation:			Knee joint: 5.1 (3–8) weeks	
			Ankle joint: 7.1 (1.5–22) weeks	
Results:				
Joints preserved:	47		Follow up:	
Amputation:	5		60 after 8.9 (2–62) months	
Arthrodesis:	6			
Resection arthropl.:	2			

Dislocations

During the same period 10 soft tissue knee injuries were managed with temporary external transfixation. Four knee joints had closed dislocations with vascular lesions, 4 had grade III open dislocations without vascular injury, and 2 had an open dislocation with vascular injury (Table 2).

A bilateral frame was applied in 4 cases, a triangular frame in 4, and a unilateral anterior half frame in 2 cases.

The mean duration of the external fixation was 6.5 (2–11) weeks. Six weeks of immobilization was considered necessary for ligamentous injuries. In 2 patients this was not possible: in 1 case infection required an arthrodesis and the other died from pulmonary embolism 2 weeks following injury. In 3 patients the fixation was maintained longer than 6 weeks due to deficiencies of soft tissue healing.

Table 2. External articular transfixation for knee dislocations. July 1974–Dec. 1982

Closed dislocation with vascular injury:			4
Grade III open dislocation without vascular injury:			4
Grade III open dislocation with vascular injury:			2
Unilateral anterior half frame:		2	
Bilateral frame:		4	
Triangular frame:		4	
Results:			
Joints preserved:	7	Follow-up:	
Arthrodesis:	1	8 after 34.6 (8–68) months	

5. Results

Fractures

After a mean follow-up of 8.9 months (2–62), 47 of the 60 patients reviewed had a functioning joint. An arthrodesis had to be performed in 6 cases, and amputation was required in 5 others. In 2 cases a resection arthroplasty of the elbow joint was performed because of infection: the resulting function was good.

The functional results will not be described in detail because of the great diversity in the type, localization, and severity of the injuries, and because a large percentage of patients had multiple trauma. Some of the patients are still undergoing treatment.

Dislocations

After a mean follow-up of 34.6 months (8–68), 7 of the 8 patients reviewed had a functioning joint. Due to infection 1 patient required an arthrodesis. In terms of joint motion and stability, the results was rated good in 6 patients and satisfactory in 1 patient. In 5 patients the joint was stable, while 2 others had an instability that was well compensated by muscular action and caused no complaints. Three patients displayed a flexion contracture of 10° or less.

Roentgenologic Changes

Only 4 knee joints and 6 ankle joints were free of roentgenologic changes after a follow-up period of at least 1 year. The remaining patients showed some deossification after the first postoperative year.

Two knee joints showed evidence of mild to moderate degenerative changes 40 and 51 months after dislocation. No such changes were seen in the ankle joints that had been immobilized with a transfixing frame, although in many of these cases only a relatively short follow-up time was available.

Since the last evaluation of cases through Dec. 1982, many additional cases of transfixations were performed until July 1983, comprising 106 fracture cases and 14 cases with knee dislocations (Table 3).

Table 3. External articular transfixation. July 1974–July 1983

Fractures:		Knee dislocations:	
Elbow joint:	6	Without vascular injury:	6
Wrist:	21	With vascular injury:	8
Hip joint:	3		
Knee:	20		
Ankle joint:	56		
	106		14

6. Discussion

External fixation is of outstanding value in the management of severe soft tissue injuries. Applied away from the injured area with a minimum of surgical trauma, the external fixator greatly facilitates the treatment of major soft tissue lesions in proximity to the joints (Rogge et al. 1980; Schmelzeisen et al. 1982). It also provides a means of stabilizing periarticular fractures that cannot be adequately immoblized by internal methods, and, in the ankle joint, it is an effective prophylactic measure against equinus deformity. The only negative points that have been expressed about external fixation relate to problems of prolonged joint immobilization with a relatively rigid system.

The regressive effect of a joint immobilization on the microstructure of the articular cartilage is well known and has been documented by a number of authors (Cotta et al. 1976; Refior et al. 1976).

Experiments in rabbits have demonstrated irreversible damage to articular cartilage, even to the point of ulceration, following a six-week period of immobilization (Finsterbush 1975). Other animal studies on the uptake of 35 S-sulphate by articular cartilage have shown that significant changes suggesting a reduced cartilage viability appear after only 4 days of immobilization (Viedman et al. 1976).

However, we feel that decades of clinical experience with conservative fracture management cast doubt on the general clinical validity of these findings in experimental animals, or at least warrant caution in their interpretation, though the major tendency of these findings certainly has to be accepted. The arguments presented do nothing to undermine the value of temporary joint immobilization with an external frame. It is reasonable to assume, in fact, that the excellent access and stability provided by the external fixator will actually shorten immobilization time compared to ordinary conservative methods and thus will reduce the probability of serious sequelae. What is more, this technique makes it possible to perform reconstructive and salvaging procedures that would be doomed to failure under conventional immobilization.

7. Conclusions

The fate of a periarticular limb injury is critically influenced by the degree of associated soft tissue trauma. Extensive soft tissue injuries require special immobilization to expedite healing and functional recovery. The external fixator, applied across the affected joint for a limited period of time, is ideally suited to meet the specific therapeutic requirements of such injuries. Any large joint may be immobilized in this fashion.

Due to varying problems of indication and management, a distinction must be made among the following types of injury:

1. Fractures with severe soft tissue injury that are amenable to stable internal fixation.
2. Fractures with severe soft tissue injury that cannot be stabilized by internal fixation alone, especially when associated with bone loss.
3. Fractures in which the extent and localization of soft tissue trauma or the fracture itself precludes internal fixation.
4. Joint disruption with severe soft tissue injury.

Temporary external articular transfixation can serve various purposes in the treatment of these injuries, depending on whether it is used to stabilized soft tissues or the bone.

Through proper and consistent application of principles and techniques described, the management of joint injuries with severe soft tissue trauma can be greatly simplified, treatment time shortened, and the functional end result improved. Applied judiciously, external articular transfixation can significantly broaden our capabilities for the repair and reconstruction of severe joint injuries.

References

1. Cotta H, Puhl W (1976) Pathophysiologie des Knorpelschadens. Hefte Unfallheilkd 127:1
2. Finsterbush A, Friedman D (1975) Reversibility of the joint changes produced by immobilization in rabbits. Clin Orthop 111:228
3. Refior HJ, Hackenbroch NH Jr (1976) Die Reaktion des hyalinen Gelenkknorpels unter Druck, Immobilisation und Distraktion. Hefte Unfallheilkd 127:23
4. Rogge D, Muhr G, Trentz O, Gotzen L (1980) Die äußere Transfixation großer Gelenke bei schwerem Weichteilschaden. Langenbecks Arch Chir 352:573
5. Schmelzeisen H, Kohler J, Packi W (1982) Gelenknahe und gelenküberbrückende Osteosynthese mit dem Fixateur externe. Akt Traumatol 12:86
6. Tscherne H, Brüggemann H (1976) Die Weichteilbehandlung bei Osteosynthesen, insbesondere bei offenen Frakturen. Unfallheilkd 79:467
7. Viedman T, Michelson JE, Rauhamäki R, Langenskjöld R (1976) Changes in 35 S-Sulphate uptake in different tissues in the knee and hip regions and rabbits during immobilization, remobilization and the development of osteoarthritis. Acta Orthop Scand 47:290

Guidelines for the Postoperative Management of Fractures with Severe Soft Tissue Injuries

E. G. Suren

1. General Principles and Goals of Postoperative Care

The main goals of the postoperative care of fractures with severe soft tissue injury are to achieve a rapid consolidation of the fracture and restore the highest level of function possible while avoiding complications. Postoperative care should be placed on the same level of importance as the operative procedure itself, for a badly-managed postoperative course can spoil the results of even the most intricate primary surgery. Consequently, the arrangement and supervision of postoperative care should be the *responsibility of the physician* and not of nursing personnel. Only the physician knows the status of his patient with regard to the injuries that have been sustained, the nature and outcome of operative treatment, and so on. This makes it essential that the attending physician have a sound grasp of the possibilities and limitations of postoperative care measures.

The first attending surgeon, in consultation with the ward physician, the physiotherapist and nursing personnel, should set up an individualized plan of postoperative care which takes into account both the overall status of the patient (age, mentality, motivation, coexisting illnesses) as well as the specifics of the injury and the kind of care that may be administered (extent of soft tissue trauma, degree of exercise or weight bearing allowed by fixation devices). This plan should not be viewed as a rigid scheme, but should be adapted as needed in the face of changes that arise during the postoperative course. This requires that close contact be maintained between the physiotherapist and the attending physician, who should not limit their participation to an occasional visit.

2. The Phases of Postoperative Care

We may identify four main phases in the postoperative care of fractures with severe soft tissue injuries:
a) The acute phase (immediate postoperative care).
b) The secondary operative phase (planned secondary procedures).
c) The functional rehabilitation phase.
d) Removal of internal fixation material.

a) Acute Phase

Dressings and Positioning. Postoperative care starts in the operating room at the time the first dressing is applied and the extremity is positioned by the surgeon. Both measures help to reduce swelling while protecting the wound from mechanical irritation. Circulation in the operative area is an important concern at this time and should be closely watched. A proven bandaging technique is to apply a layer of sterile cotton padding over the sterile wound dressing and then apply a rolled-on elastic bandage under moderate pressure to limit swelling. This bandage, as well as any plaster fixation that may be required, is *applied only after the extremity has been placed in the definitive postoperative position* judged to be most favorable in a functional sense. This is necessary to avoid constrictions and associated pressure lesions (Fig. 1).

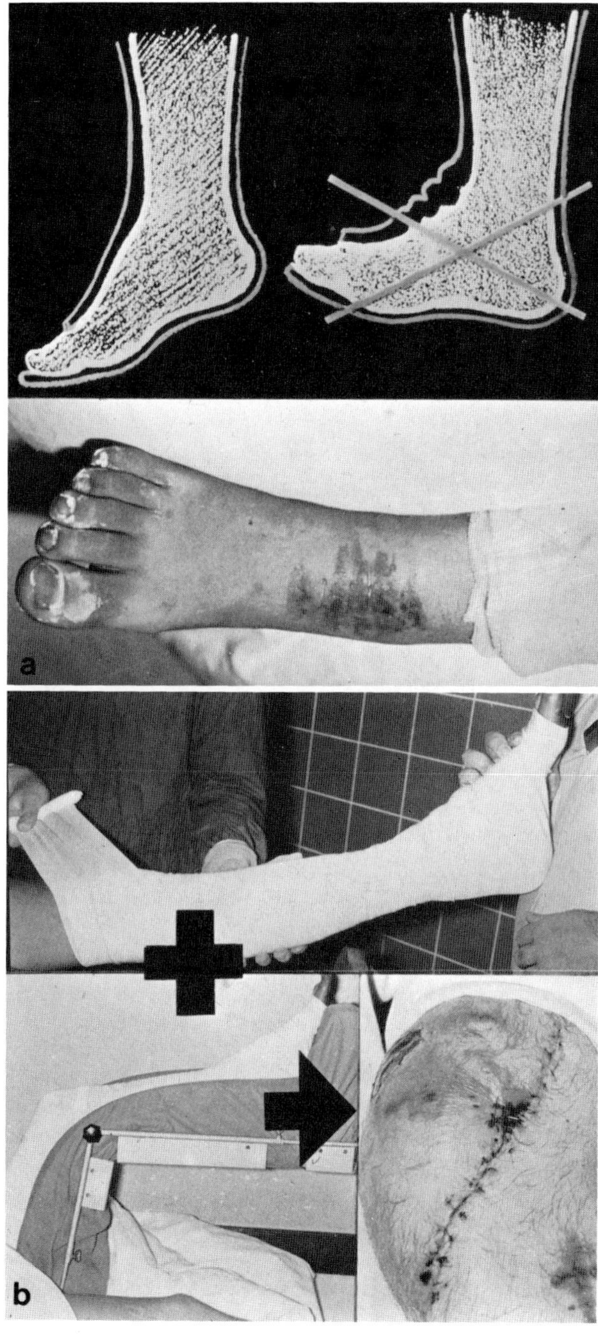

Fig. 1. a The plaster immobilization of a joint in an unphysiologic position can lead to creasing and lesions of the soft tissue. **b** Bandaging the knee joint in extension and then flexing it over a 90° splint causes pressure necrosis of the soft tissues over the patella

Suspension of the extremity is useful in facilitating care of the operative area (e.g., in the presence of circumferential skin loss). The suspension rig may be attached to a previously applied external frame or to Kirschner wires inserted temporarily for that purpose. *Forced elevation is inappropriate,* as it may compromise blood flow to the traumatized soft tissues. If soft tissue conditions are precarious, or if an impending or manifest compartment syndrome is present, the extremity should be elevated no higher than 10 cm above the level of the atria.

Positioning Splints. Postoperative positioning in conventional splints can sometimes be troublesome, especially in polytrauma patients. In the lower extremity, foam splints that extend the full length of the leg can compromise venous return in the thigh and predispose to thrombosis, especially in obese individuals. They can also promote flexion contractures of the hip and knee joint when their use is prolonged.

Poorly-fitting foam splints whose diameter does not conform to that of the extremity interfere with circulation and may allow unacceptable pressure to be placed on soft tissues and nerves (e.g., at the head of the fibula). In an effort to reduce the difficulties of post-

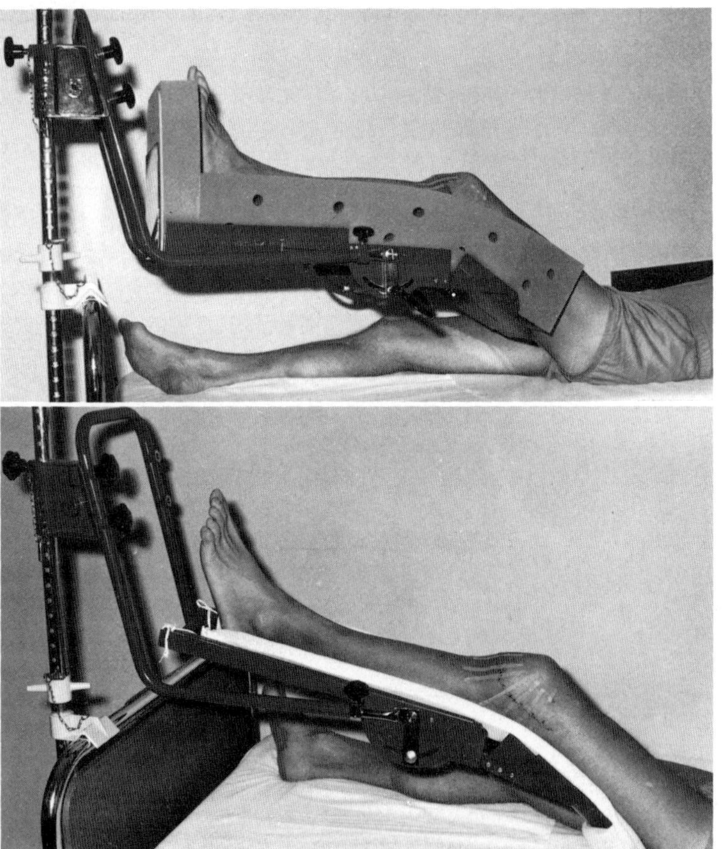

Fig. 2. Adjustable splint developed at the Trauma Center of Hannover Medical School for postoperative positioning of the lower extremity (Giebel, Tscherne 1981)

operative lower-extremity elevation, two new splints have been developed at our hospital (Giebel, Tscherne 1981) which combine the advantages of stable positioning in a foam-padded elevation splint with the ease of access and accurate fit of the free-hanging Krapp splint (Fig. 2).

Errors and Hazards. In the acute phase it is imperative that *circulation, sensation and motility* be checked at regular intervals by the physican and nursing personnel. If circulatory conditions are uncertain or precarious at operation, the elastic bandage applied postoperatively should be slit for its entire length after 2–4 hours as a preventive measure against compartment syndrome. This is particularly important in children, especially following internal fixations in the elbow region, and in elderly, cerebrosclerotic patients.

During routine postoperative visits, the physician and nursing personnel should be alert for *errors of positioning,* especially following operations under spinal anesthesia, so that pressure injury to nerves and soft tissues can be avoided.

In addition, nursing personnel should watch for the *warning signals of circulatory impairment or nerve injury,* which are listed in Table 1. It is important that nurses be familiar with these warning signals and notify the physician at once of their occurrence, day or night, so that prompt, specific action can be taken. Waiting constitutes gross negligence that may result in loss of disability of the limb.

Table 1. Warning signals of complications in the acute postoperative phase

1. Persistent or increasing pain
2. Redness, heat, swelling
3. Paresthesias
4. Restricted motion in the fingers or toes
5. Temperature differences (especially of the extremities)
6. Pathologic discolorations (especially of the extremities): pale white, livid

Drug Therapy to Improve Peripheral Flow. If the circulatory status of large, crushed skin areas is equivocal at operation, the intravenous injection of low molecular weight dextran and the administration of bupivacaine (0.25%) by *peridural catheter* may occasionally be indicated. The latter increases blood flow through its sympathicolyte action while also decreasing pain during the immediate postoperative period. The peridural catheter may be left in place for 1–2 weeks if meticulous care is maintained.

Postoperative Physiotherapy. While *early postoperative mobilization* is a fundamental principle in the internal fixation of fractures, it is not generally advised for fractures associated with severe soft tissue injury because of its potentially detrimental effect on wound healing. However, there are cases in which controlled exercises performed from a split cast may be allowed if no complications are present and the fracture has been stably immobilized. The decision rests with the surgeon. Only he can accurately assess the status of the soft tissues, bone and internal fixation and weigh the risks accordingly. In any case, the need to await soft tissue healing does not mean that the patient should be inactive postoperatively. Even with a massively traumatized limb, much benefit can be derived from *Böhler's classic guidelines for postoperative fracture care* (1943).

In addition to active movements of all noninjured and nonimmobilized joints, emphasis is placed upon regular isometric exercises of the injured extremity as a means of improving circulation and preventing swelling and thromboembolic disease. Thus, the physiotherapist is called in at a relatively early stage.

Thromboembolic Prophylaxis. Special attention should be given to the prevention of thromboembolic complications during postoperative care, particularly since the ^{125}I-fibrinogen test has demonstrated deep venous thrombosis in up to 47% of patients who have undergone trauma surgery (Nicolaides 1972). Besides the usual risk factors, the nature, extent, duration and localization of the trauma or surgery play a significant role in the pathogenesis of thromboembolism. The thrombogenic "triad" described by Virchow in 1856 is a common occurrence in accident victims with severe tissue trauma (Tables 2 and 3).

For this reason, all bed-confined patients at our hospital are placed on a rigorous program of thromboembolic prophylaxis which involves a combination of mechanical, physiotherapeutic and pharmacologic measures. The foremost *mechanical measures* are a stable operative fixation of the fracture and the application of compression stockings. Also, on the day of the operation the physiotherapist institutes *general physiotherapeutic measures* which include *isometric exercises of the injured extremity* and *active range-of-motion*

Table 2. Thrombotic risk factors

General	Trauma, Surgery
1. Age	depends on:
2. Cardiovascular disease	1. Localization
3. Vasopathy (e.g., varicosities)	2. Nature
4. Obesity	3. Extent
5. Contraceptives	4. Duration
6. Inactivity	

Table 3. Virchow's triad of thrombogenesis

1. *Stasis*
Post-traumatic swelling
Postop. immobilization
2. *Hypercoagulability*
Tissue trauma
3. *Vessel wall lesions*
Traumatic
Ischemic

exercises for all uninjured joints. The patient must be suitably instructed and motivated so that he will be able to perform these exercises by himself at regular intervals.

We also prescribe low-dose heparinization (5000 U b.i.d. or t.i.d.) for all bed-confined patients over 16 years of age, including those with polytrauma. This regimen is continued until ambulation is possible (Table 4).

Table 4. Prophylaxis of postoperative thromboembolism

1. Mechanical measures
Special bilateral leg bandages (elastic)
Bilateral compression stockings
Pneumatic alternating-pressure boots
Stable operative fixation of fracture
2. Physiotherapeutic measures
Isometric exercises
Respiratory exercises
Active exercises
3. Pharmacologic measures
Low-dose heparin (2–3 x 5000 U/day)

b) Secondary Operative Phase

If the condition of the soft tissues is satisfactory at the end of the acute phase, planned secondary procedures may be carried out. These consist essentially of definitive wound closure, additional stabilization of the fracture, and the repair of osseous defects.

Definitive Wound Closure. Wounds covered primarily with synthetic skin dressing require close supervision with regular dressing changes at 2- to 3-day intervals. If no residual devitalization or infection is noted, then the wound may be approximated in stages with sterile adhesive strips, closed by secondary suture, or covered with a meshed split-thickness skin graft.

Wounds with tissue loss and pocketing are highly susceptible to hematoma formation and infection under a dressing. It is important, therefore, that the synthetic skin be accurately molded to wound contours when applied so that maximal contact is obtained. A light pressure stint made of foam rubber or gauze may also be applied if desired. Daily synthetic skin changes and wound inspection are basic in managing problem wounds of this type.

The size of the soft tissue defect requiring closure is partly influenced by the *bandaging technique* used in the postoperative period. After acute swelling has subsided, the muscles have a tendency to sag (especially in the lower leg) and should be held up by an elastic bandage wrapped around the limb under moderate pressure so that wound size can be reduced. When dealing with extensive soft tissue defects and problem wounds, especially those over exposed bone, *reconstructive plastic surgery* is indicated (Table 5).

A meshed split-thickness skin graft is useful for providing the clean wound conditions that are a prerequisite for these technically complex reconstructive techniques.

Table 5. Possibilities for the definitive closure of problem wounds

1. Advancement flaps
2. Myogenic flaps
3. Myocutaneous flaps
4. Cross-leg flaps
5. Microvascular free flaps

Stabilization of the Fracture. Circumstances may warrant a *change in the method of fracture stabilization* during the postoperative period. Hence, the attending physician must have a thorough understanding of the options that are available in any given situation and how they might influence osseous blood flow in fractures with severe soft tissue injury (Table 6).

For example, an external fixation frame may be removed from the leg and replaced with a walking cast once the wound has been definitively closed and there is early evidence of fracture consolidation. In fractures that have been stabilized by compression plating, the application of an external frame may be indicated if infection or instability arises. Plates used to bidge long osseous defects, especially in the tibia, can be stabilized externally by applying a half frame comparily.

We reject the notion of "minimal internal fixation" in the primary care of fractures with severe soft tissue injury, due to the inherent instability of such techniques. The true goal should be a *stable internal fixation with a minimum of implanted material.* If circumstances do not permit a stable internal fixation to be performed primarily, it should be done secondarily as soon as possible, since stability is the best safeguard against infection.

Table 6. Options for chancing the modality of fracture fixation

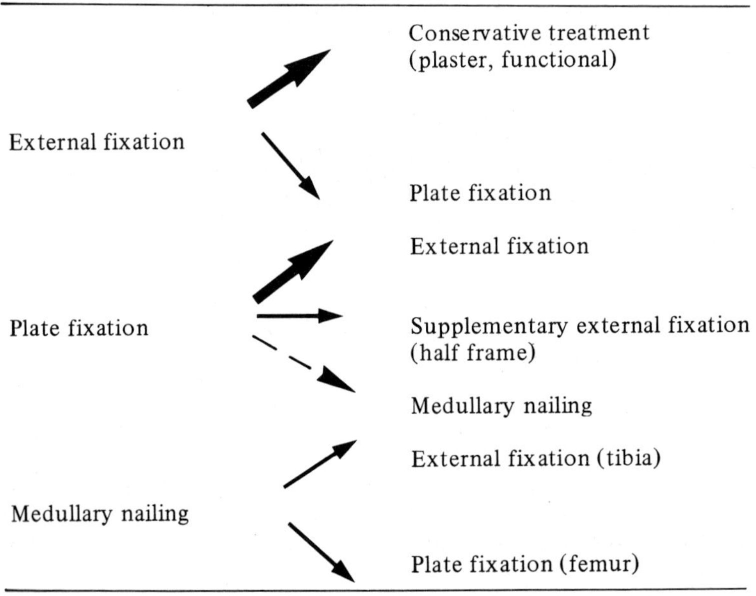

Repair of Osseous Defects. The successful primary repair of bone defects requires accurate planning and a high level of experience on the part of the surgeon. Additional prerequisites are a good soft-tissue environment, a well-perfused recipient bed, a stable fixation, and a patient who will remain cooperative during a lengthy and sometimes arduous convalescence. In cerebrosclerotic patients, alcoholics, and patients with a poor social background, the surgical repair of an extensive bone defect is doomed to failure from the outset, and therefore is contraindicated. The defect may be filled with autologous cancellous bone or corticocancellous grafts. A small degree of limb shortening may occur and is considered an acceptable byproduct of the procedure (Fig. 3).

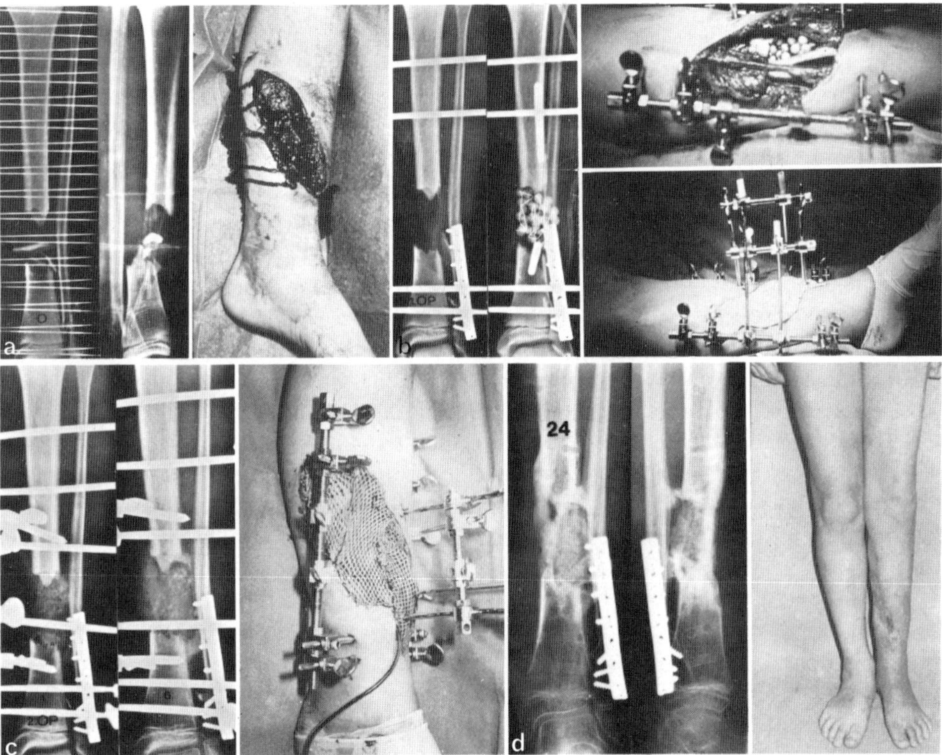

Fig. 3. a Grade III open tibial fracture with bone loss and lacerated posterior tibial artery in an 11-year-old boy. **b** One hour postinjury the wound was debrided and an external frame applied, resulting in a 2-cm shortening of the limb. The fibula was plated to enhance stability. The osseous defect was packed primarily with PMMA beads as a prelude to secondary cancellous grafting. The shortening enabled a tension-free muscle coverage to be obtained. The wound was temporarily covered with Epigard. **c** The postoperative course was uneventful, and 1 week later a 2nd operation was performed in which the osseous defect was filled with autologous cancellous bone and a meshed split-thickness skin graft was applied. **d** Six weeks postinjury the external frame was removed and an above-knee walking cast was applied. At 16 weeks bone healing was satisfacotry and the cast was removed. A full-weight-bearing orthosis was prescribed for 1 year. The radiographic and external appearance of the operated limb after 24 weeks are shown

Microvascular bone transfers (e.g., from the fibula, rib or iliac crest) are reserved for selected cases and specialized centers.

c) Functional Rehabilitation Phase

The final goal of postoperative care is functional rehabilitation, i.e., returning the injured limb to function while returning the patient to a productive existence. This phase of postoperative care differs little from that which follows the internal fixation of closed fractures (Table 7).

Table 7. The stages of functional rehabilitation

1. Physio therapy, mobilization, ambulation training
2. Assisted exercises (active, motion splint)
3. Incremental weight bearing
4. Assistive orthopedic devices (e.g., orthoses)
5. Vocational rehabilitation

Functional rehabilitation is accomplished chiefly through *therapeutic exercises performed actively and without force or pain.* Given the disturbances of osseous blood flow and bone healing that are characteristic of fractures with severe soft tissue injury, the lower extremity will require a *protracted period of non-weight bearing* with active exercise of the foot (alternating dorsiflexion and plantar flexion). Graduated weight bearing may be instituted in accordance with roentgenologic findings and soft tissue healing.

In fractures of the lower extremity (especially intraarticular fractures) that are fixed securely enough to permit exercise, *continuous passive mobilization on a motion splint* has proven beneficial in cases where soft tissue status is good (Fig. 4). The constant pattern of alternating loads promotes nutrition of the articular cartilage and discourages the development of intra-articular adhesions and contractures. The range of motion through which the joint is taken should be closely watched by the surgeon and modified as needed according to soft tissue healing and the stability of the fixation. A valuable index is the patient's pain threshold, which should just be reached with each stress increment. *Icing* of the operated limb is an excellent means of raising the pain threshold.

Following fractures of the lower leg with extensive devascularisation of the bone, following repair of large osseous defects and in tibia fractures with consecutive osteitis which needed sequestrotomy and bone grafting an orthosis should be prescribed after removal of an external fixator to avoid refractures and fatique fractures. This device will allow full axial weight bearing while protecting the lower leg from bending stress.

d) Removal of Internal Fixation Material

In fractures with severe soft tissue trauma, plates should be left in place for at least 2 to 2 1/2 years due to the significant impairment of osseous blood flow. The plates may be removed only after clear roentgenologic evidence of consolidation has been obtained (verified if necessary by special views). When removing the plate, care should be taken not to remove the bony ridges that have formed around the plate margins, because they provide added stability. In fractures of this type that are associated with disturbances of osseous

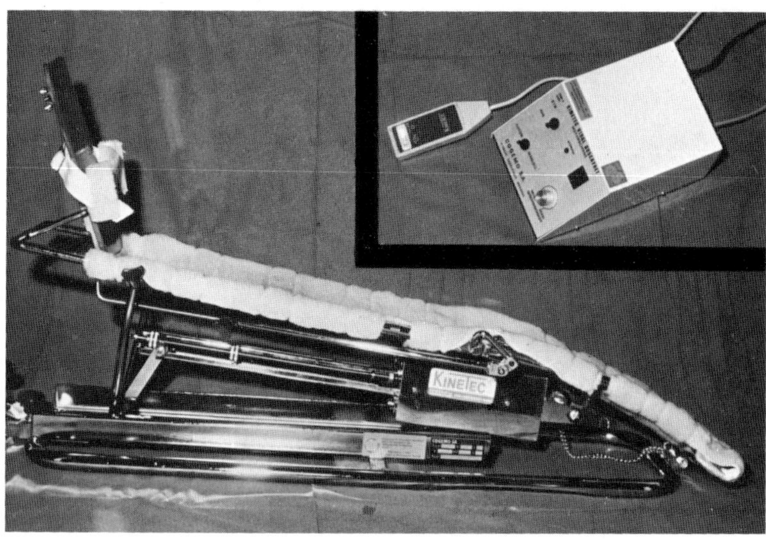

Fig. 4. Automatic passive motion splint which can be set to any speed and range of motion desired

blood flow, the patient should bear weight cautiously for at least two months following implant removal and should refrain from sporting activities for at least six months as a precaution against refracture.

The following case report is presented to illustrate the various stages of postoperative care (Fig. 5):

A motorcyclist who was struck directly in the leg by the bumper of a truck presented with a grade III open supracondylar and diacondylar fracture of the femur with comminution of the lateral condyle, an open knee joint, a grade III open comminuted fracture of the distal tibia, and extensive degloving of soft tissues (Fig. 5a).

Primary care was administered within 3 hours postinjury. The soft tissues were extensively debrided, an emergency four-compartment fasciotomy was performed in the lower leg, and an external frame was applied across the ankle joint. The distal fibula was plated to improve stability (Fig. 5b).

The articular surface of the femur was reconstructed and fixed with a condylar buttress plate and lag screws. An external frame was applied temporarily across the knee joint to remove stress from the internal fixation and facilitate nursing care; plaster fixation was not used (Fig. 5c and d).

When local heat and slight redness were noted in the knee on the 3rd postoperative day, the patient was returned to OR for a second look, at which time demarcated areas of soft tissue necrosis were found and widely excised. Cultured smears from the wound were negative. The skin at the knee was closed by secondary suture, and meshed grafts were applied to the distal thigh. Isometric muscle-strengthening exercises were initiated.

Postoperative course was uneventful, and in the 3rd week a 3rd operation was performed in which osseous defects in the distal femur were packed with autologous cancellous bone (Fig. 5d). In week 4 the external articular transfixation was removed from the knee. Passive mobilization was started on a motion splint (Fig. 5e), and non-weight bearing ambulation was also initiated.

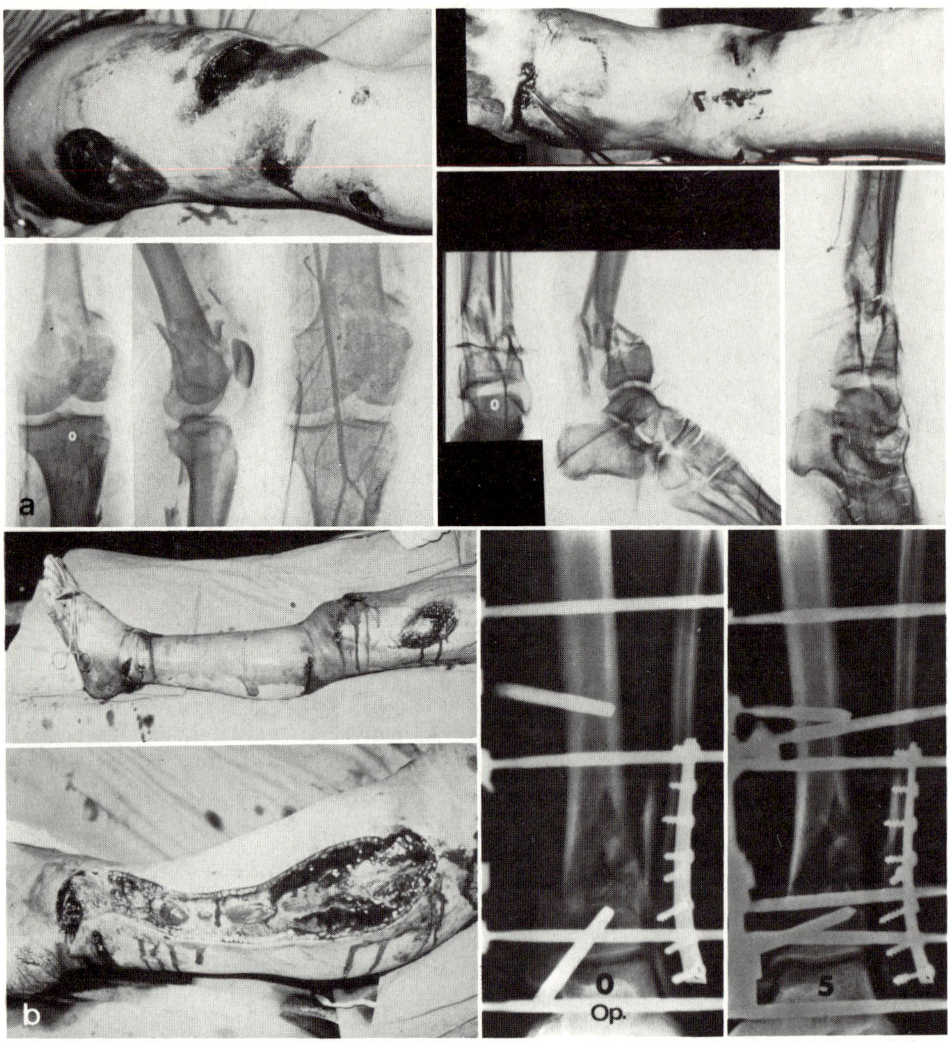

Fig. 5a–b. (See text)

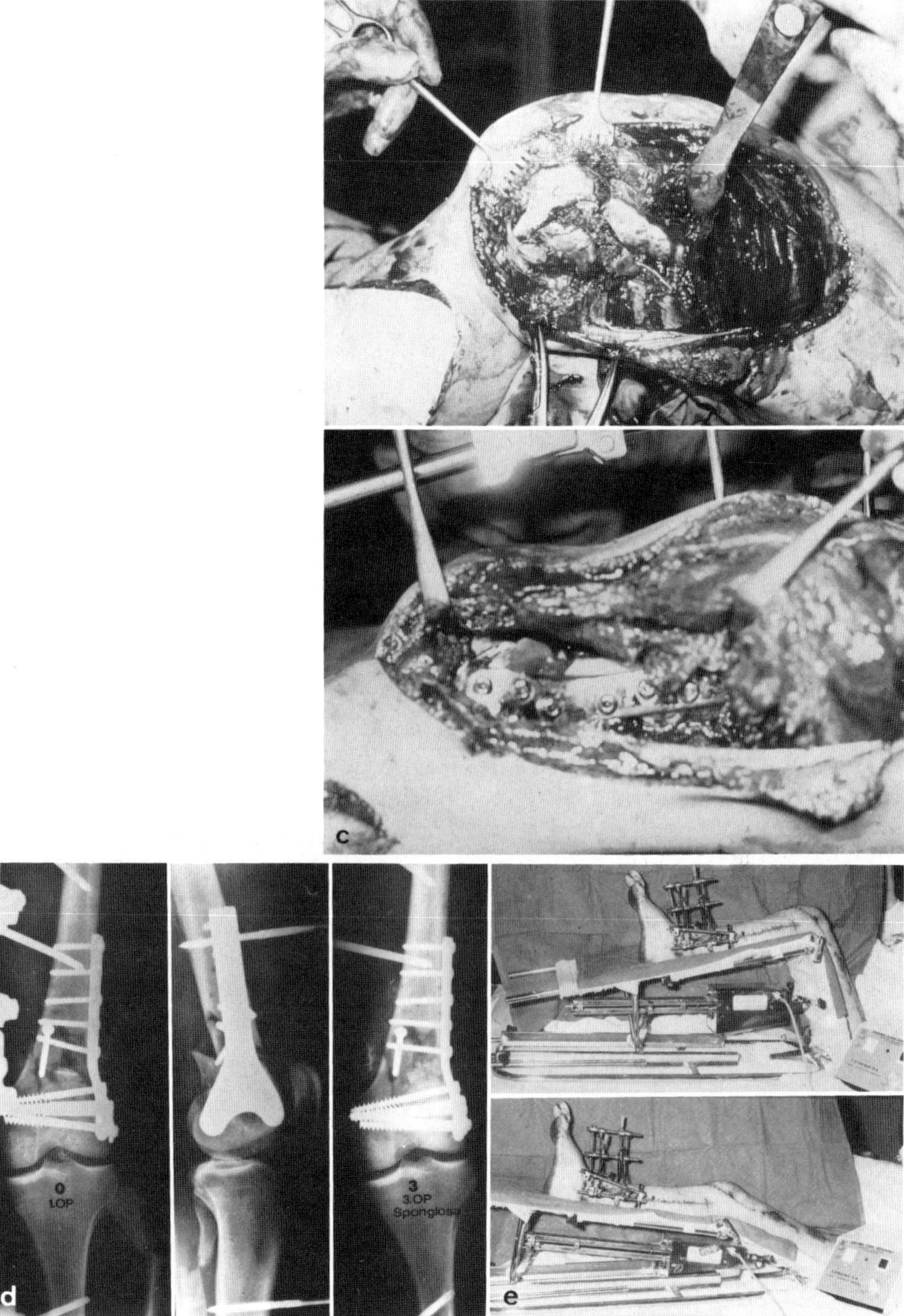

Fig. 5c–e. (See text)

3. Conclusions

The postoperative care of fractures with severe soft tissue injuries requires close teamwork between the traumatologist, physiotherapist and nursing personnel. It requires a deep commitment from all parties involved, including the patient. "Loving care" and idleness are of no benefit. Only a rigorous yet flexible program of postoperative care *and* suitable patient guidance can produce the desired result: a full recovery of function.

References

1. Böhler L (1943) Die Technik der Knochenbruchbehandlung. Maudrich, Wien
2. Friedrich B (1979) Die funktionelle Nachbehandlung von Osteosynthesen. Chirurg 50:742
3. Giebel G, Tscherne H (1981) Die Lagerung der unteren Extremität – Ein neues Schienenprogramm –. Chirurg 52:791
4. List M (1979) Zur Nachbehandlung von Patienten mit Osteosynthesen aus krankengymnastischer Sicht. Chirurg 50:746
5. Müller HJ (1978) Frühfunktionelle Behandlung der Problemfrakturen nach Osteosynthesen. Schriften Unfallmed Tag d gewerbl Berufsgenossenschaften 34:51
6. Müller HJ (1979) Übungsbehandlung nach Osteosynthesen aus ärztlicher Sicht. Chirurg 50:739
7. Nikolaides AN et al. (1972) Small doses of subcutaneous sodium heparin in preventing deep venous thrombosis after major surgery. Lancet 890
8. Petracic B (1979) Funktionelle Nachbehandlung operierter Knochenbrüche. Thieme, Stuttgart
9. Rube R (1981) Kryotherapie in der physikalischen Medizin. Z Allg Med 57:2411
10. Rüedi Th, Allgöwer M (1975) Richtlinien der Schweizerischen AO für die Nachbehandlung operativ versorgter Frakturen. AO-Bulletin
11. Schlegel KF (1979) Die krankengymnastische, physikalische und beschäftigungstherapeutische Begleitbehandlung von Verletzungen in der Frühphase. Hefte Unfallheikd 138:232
12. Schmidt HG, Morgenroth B (1980) Zusammenarbeit von Arzt, Therapeut und Handwerker nach Osteosynthesen. Schriftenr Unfallmed Tag d gewerbl Berufsgenossenschaften 40:115
13. Schweickert CH (1971) Fehler in der Nachbehandlung. Langenbecks Arch Chir 329: 1152
14. Suren EG, Kunert P (1981) Nachbehandlungsprinzipien bei Handverletzungen. Chirurg 52:210
15. Tscherne H, Westermann K, Trentz O, Pretschner P, Mellmann J (1978) Thromboembolische Komplikationen und ihre Prophylaxe beim Hüftgelenkersatz. Unfallheilkd 81:178
16. Tscherne H (1971) Die Nachbehandlung operierter Knochenbrüche. Wiener Med Wschr 3:38
17. Tscherne H, Deutsch E (1981) Postoperative Thromboembolieprophylaxe aus aktueller Sicht. Thieme, Stuttgart
18. Virchow R (1856) Gesammelte Abhandlungen zur wissenschaftlichen Medizin. Meidinger u. Sohn, Frankfurt

Early Complications of Fractures with Soft Tissue Injuries

G. Muhr

Early postfracture complications generally occur as a result of soft tissue damage. Necrosis, circulatory insufficiency and contamination are the main traumatic or iatrogenic factors which precipitate complications. Frequently they are compounded by the trauma-related shock. While these factors are qualitatively present in any soft tissue injury, it is their quantitative extent which ultimately is responsible for complications. Thus, preventive therapy consists in preserving or restoring blood flow to the soft tissues by controlling shock and alleviating local pathogenic factors such as fragment pressure, tissue edema and compartment syndrome. If the wound is presumed to be contaminated, these measures are supplemented by meticulous debridement and antibiotic therapy.

The major early complications of fractures with soft tissue injury are as follows:

1. Necrosis of Skin and Soft Tissues

Foci of contusion are a very common nidus for soft tissue necrosis. The true extent of the necrosis is difficult to determine initially, because local or general blood flow disturbances compound the damage. Mechanical or metabolic edema with acidosis leads to thrombosis of the marginal blood vessels, and the necrosis spreads. A similar situation is seen in degloving injuries, which are almost invariably associated with extensive necrosis of the avulsed skin.

The contusional necrosis is not amenable to treatment. However, its spread can be controlled by preserving the blood flow to peripheral tissues (decompressing the soft tissues, stabilizing the fracture, treating for edema).

Sites of full-thickness skin necrosis over soft tissues are excised after a few days, and the defect is covered with split-thickness skin. If the necrosis is located over bone, one may await granulation tissue formation under the eschar and then cover the granulating surface with split-thickness skin (Fig. 1). If early excision is necessary (e.g., because of infection), the resulting defect and exposed bone can be covered by reconstructive surgery (local or distant soft tissue flaps, free grafts).

In extensive subcutaneous degloving injuries, it is advantageous to excise the avulsed flap, defat it, and reapply it as a meshed graft either primarily or secondarily after a period of refrigerated storage (Fig. 2).

The postexcision defects are covered with synthetic skin or, if contamination is heavy, with moist, antiseptic dressings until plastic surgery can be undertaken.

Skin and soft tissue necroses associated with fracture instability are managed like an infected fracture, i.e., by wound debridement and protective fixation. The lower leg is a site of predilection for soft tissue necrosis, and external fixation is the modality of choice in such cases. If exposed bone is visible following the debridement, early plastic surgery

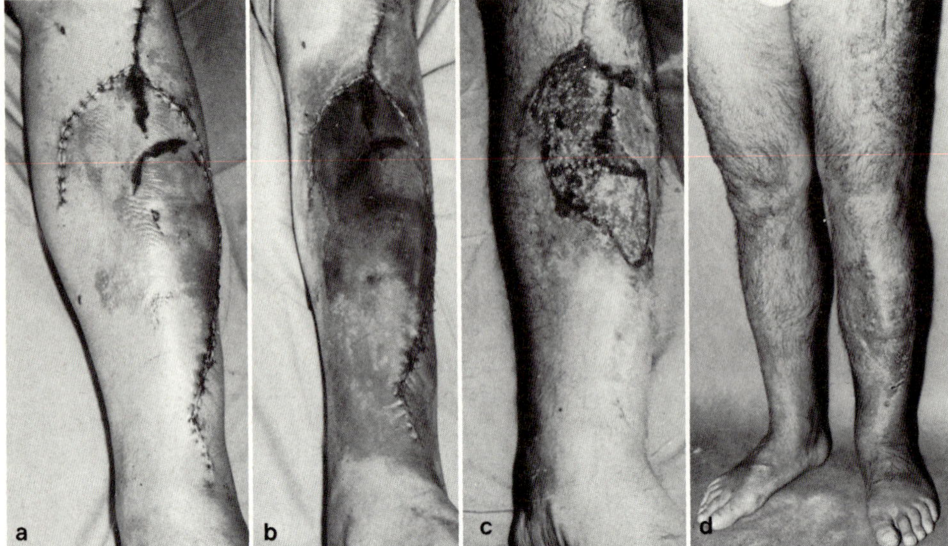

Fig. 1a–d. Open tibial fracture with full-thickness skin contusion as it appeared after internal plating (**a**). A full-thickness skin necrosis developed on the anteromedial side of the limb (**b**). A granulating surface was allowed to form, and this was subsequently covered with split-thickness skin (**c, d**)

can provide a robust integument and so is preferred over granulation healing and split-thickness skin grafting (Fig. 3).

2. Rebound Compartment Syndrome

Despite the prompt recognition and surgical treatment of a compartment syndrome, the posttraumatic and postoperative swelling that occurs within 6–12 hours can lead to development of a *rebound compartment syndrome.* Thus, peripheral neurology and blood flow should be closely monitored for 48 hours following a fasciotomy. If a rebound compartment syndrome is suspected, the overlying skin is incised at one, and the fascia and retinacula are inspected to make sure they have been adequately incised or divided. The incisions are made without regard for cosmesis, and closure is done secondarily.

3. Hematomas

The importance of post-traumatic and postoperative *hematomas* as an early fracture complication is not generally appreciated. As in other complications, the cause is traumatic or iatrogenic soft tissue injury with damage to multiple blood vessels, allowing extravasation to occur once the circulatory status has improved. Osseous vessels that have been injured by the fracture or by internal fixation (e.g., medullary nailing) may also bleed heavily.

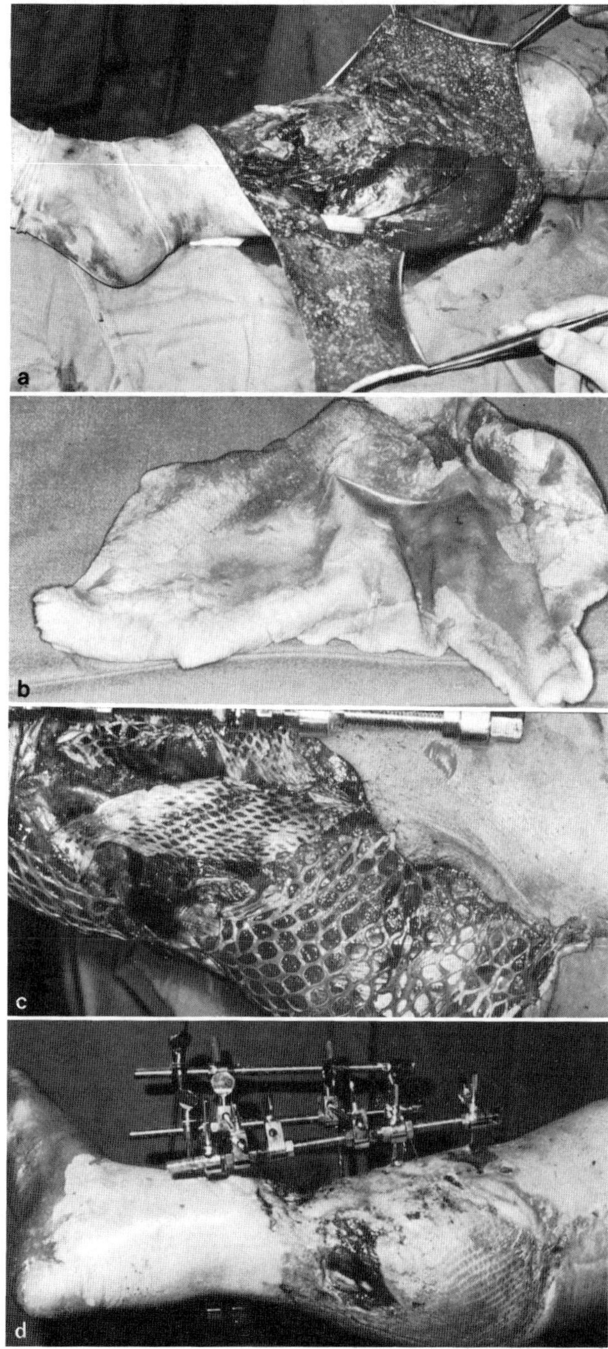

Fig. 2a–d. Grade III open tibial fracture with extensive degloving of the skin and subcutaneous tissue (**a**). The avulsed flap was excised, defatted and preserved by refrigeration (**b**). Three weeks later it was reimplanted as a meshed graft (**c**), and uneventful healing ensued (**d**)

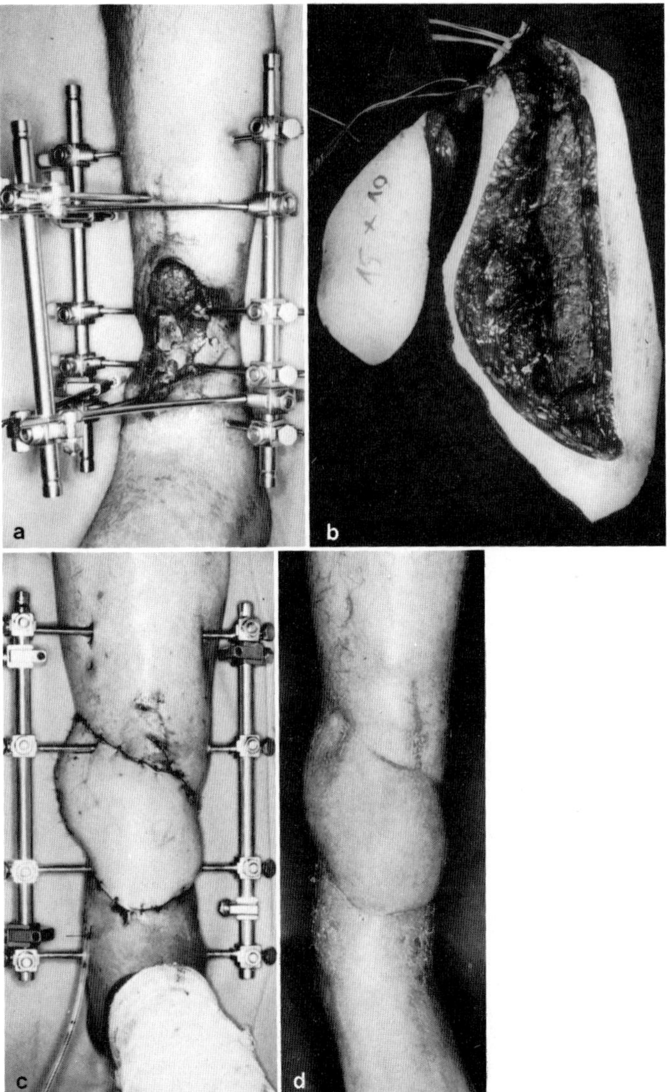

Fig. 3a–d. Open fracture of the distal tibia with large soft tissue defect and exposed bone following skin necrosis and infection (**a**). The defect was covered with a microvascular free flap (**b**, **c**), with a good end result (**d**)

Additional causes are deficient surgical hemostasis and the presence of dead spaces in the tissue.

When a postoperative hematoma is diagnosed, a wait-and-see approach is completely inappropriate, because about one-fifth of all such hematomas are presumed to be contaminated. Small, superficial hematomas are removed by aspiration: After disinfecting the skin, a local anesthetic is administered intracutaneously, and the hematoma is aspirated with a large-gauge needle introduced through a stab incision.

If blood effusions are recurrent or if hematomas are deep or extensive, the wound must be reopened under sterile operating room conditions to permit evacuation of the hematoma. Areas of subcutaneous and muscular necrosis will be apparent on exploration and must be excised. At the same time, smears are taken from the wound for cultering. Following multiple irrigations, drains are inserted, and the wound is closed without tension (otherwise secondarily).

Hemorrhagic effusions in joints are removed by percutaneous aspiration or open evacuation. If the effusion recurs, it is assumed that a traumatic synovitis is present, and anti-inflammatory therapy is indicated (drugs, icing). Even if a positive culture is obtained, continuous passive mobilization may still be carried out under an antibiotic screen (synovial pump). Hematomas should never be expressed through loosened skin sutures, and one should never await a spontaneous rupture between sutures of the operative wound. The risk of infection in such circumstances is very high, and an emergency revision is indicated.

4. Arterial and Venous Blood Flow Disturbances

Monitoring of the peripheral blood flow is basic to fracture management. Besides sensory and motor function, the peripheral pulses should always be checked before and after the fracture is reduced. This does not preclude the occurrence of secondary *arterial or venous blood flow disturbances,* however.

Acute post-traumatic circulatory disturbances are not difficult to recognize. Arterial thrombosis, on the other hand, occurs as a secondary complication and so is easily overlooked. Lesions of the intima or media which do not immediately disrupt the internal continuity of the blood vessel form a nidus for cumulative platelet aggregation, leading secondarily to the complete blockage of the vessel. A similar effect is produced by constant or intermittent pressure from bone fragments. The situation is difficult to diagnose, particularly if the patient has sustained multiple injuries and displays hemodynamic instability. In young patients there is the potential for a compensatory collateral circulation to develop, thus preventing or delaying clinical manifestations of the impaired peripheral flow (Fig. 4).

Venous embarrassment is a common phenomenon in the lower extremity. Fractures of the tibia are frequently associated with deep venous ruptures, and the venous complex may become compressed by bone fragments or hematomas. Less than one-third of patients with angiographic evidence of deep venous thrombosis display clinical symptoms. Although nearly half of all pulmonary embolisms occur within the first 2 weeks after the trauma, fatal attacks may occur until 3–4 months later.

The effects of venous stasis, which plays a significant role in the etiology of deep venous thromboses, should be taken into account in all complicated fractures. Their prevention has already been discussed (see p. 122).

When confronted with a frank deep thrombosis confirmed by phlebography, the physician should order full heparinization without delay. With thrombosis of the iliofemoral or axillary veins, thrombolytic therapy should be instituted unless a surgical thrombectomy is not indicated.

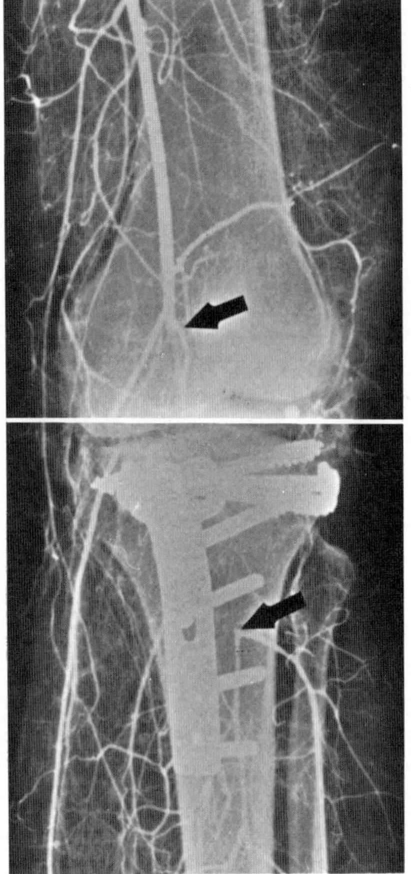

Fig. 4. Post-traumatic thrombosis of the popliteal artery secondary to a fracture-dislocation of the upper tibia. Diagnosis was delayed due to good collateralization

5. Infection

The most serious and dreaded complication of fractures is *infection.* Despite a declining prevalence and improved recovery rates with functional sequelae, the very duration of the illness, necessitating prolonged hospitalization and the loss of private and professional contacts, places a severe burden upon the patient.

The special pathophysiology of soft tissue injury with local circulatory impairment due to trauma and tissue shock, widely distended tissue spaces, and the consequent reparative inflammation create conditions that are ideal for the development of an infection. It is a short step from an open, contaminated fracture to an acute infection, whose occurrence depends quantitatively on the extent of tissue necrosis and qualitatively on the cirulence of the contaminating organisms. Thus fractures which have received inadequate primary soft tissue care must be regarded as potentially infected. Errors of treatment compound the preexisting injury.

If, following primary care, the wound is treated open and dressings are changed daily, the presence of necrosis or infection is readily confirmed at any time. Even when the skin has been closed, there should be no hesitation about reopening the wound if conditions warrant it. Increasing discharges from drains or through suture lines, local skin redness, and painful edema are symptoms of infection that are confirmed by an elevated temperature, leukocytosis and a rising ESR.

Only immediate reintervention prompted by the mere suspicion of an infection can forestall a complicated course.

Synthetic skin products (e.g., Epigard) should be applied only to smooth, uncontaminated wound surfaces. If the level of contamination is high and the wound surface is deeply pitted, aseptic dressings are preferred in the initial phase.

Extensive primary soft tissue destruction, with its associated high infection risk, is an automatic indication for a second look within 24–48 hours. Time and again we are surprised by the amount of necrotic tissue that is found at revision and by the rapid normalization of limb trophism after that tissue is excised.

6. Instability

The stability provided by the fixation device should be checked during all revisional operations. Unstable, mobile fragments tend to pump superficial wound infection into fracture

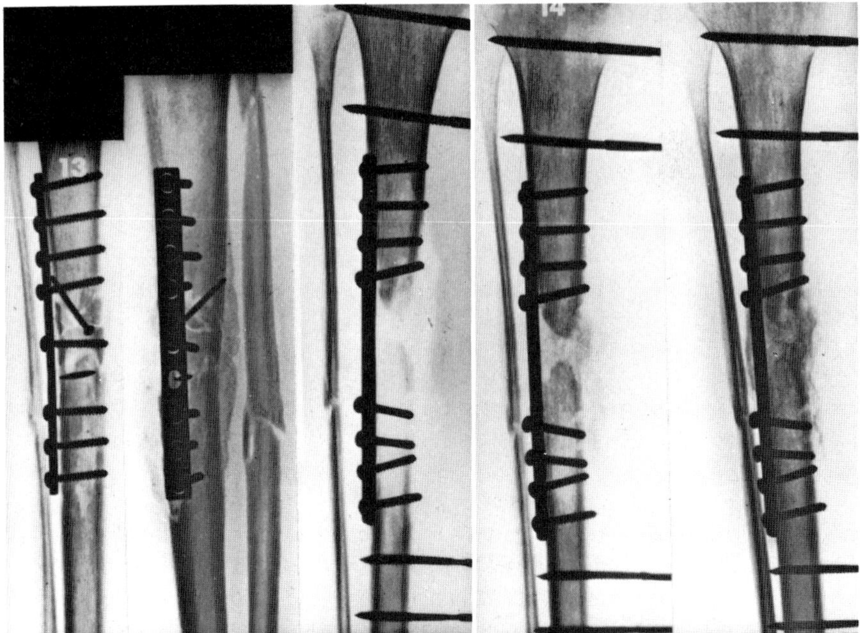

Fig. 5. Infection and plate loosening following internal fixation of an open tibial fracture. Replating was carried out and was supplemented by external half frame fixation and cancellous bone grafting. The fracture went on to uneventful union

lines and the medullary cavity, leading to osteitis. The loose implant acts as a foreign body which interferes with reparative processes, and the instability leads to disturbances of microvascularization and to osteonecrosis.

The manner of revising the failed fixation depends, in the uninfected fracture, on the nature of the primary fixation and the degree of instability present. An unstable plate fixation may be revised by replating the fracture, adding a supplementary external half frame (Fig. 5), or by applying an external fixator. If an external fixator was applied primarily, instability is easily corrected by supplementing or extending the montage, possibly adopting a joint transfixation configuration. If necessary the extremity can be suspended by the fixation rods to allow circumferential wound care.

Fractures with soft tissue injuries are highly suspectible to early complications induced by traumatic or iatrogenic embarrassment of soft tissue perfusion. The best protection against healing disturbances with their often serious consequences and poor end result is the preservation of tissue blood flow through prompt, active intervention.

The Plastic Repair of Large Soft Tissue Defects

A. Berger

1. Introduction

Large soft tissue defects produced by trauma place high demands on the skills of the operator and call for a well-defined therapeutic concept. Management becomes especially difficult when the soft tissue defects are combined with a bone fracture. The basic approach in such cases is to render expert primary care that will establish a sound basis for subsequent reconstructive surgery. The main priority of primary care is the avoidance of infection.

The first step in treatment is to inspect the injury to ascertain its nature, and espcially its depth. The second step is a radical wound debridement to remove all crushed and contaminated tissues. The true depth of the soft tissue wound can be accurately assessed at that time. As a third step, the osseous injury is stabilized using any of the various fixation methods available (described elsewhere in this volume). The final step is coverage of the soft tissue defect.

The strategy for procuring soft tissue coverage is influenced by the degree of exposure of bone, tendons and nerves. Bone that is devoid of periosteum requires coverage with a fat-dermis flap, fascia or muscle. Exposed nerves and tendons should likewise be covered with a soft tissue mantle possessing a good blood supply.

Superficial skin and soft tissue defects may be closed primarily by split-thickness skin grafting. This procedure must be integrated into the overall plan of treatment. If it is not possible to procure coverage of exposed bone, tendons and nerves during primary care, then early secondary grafting should be untertaken within a few days.

Split-Thickness Skin Grafts

In defects with a good wound bed, primary split-thickness skin grafting may be utilized. The use of a fenestrated graft with a mesh ratio of 1 : 1.5 to 1 :3 is the method of choice, as this type of graft is best to tolerate postoperative edema and bleeding. Because the wound area, wound bed and course of healing cannot always be accurately assessed primarily, it is best to cover the wound temporarily with a synthetic skin dressing and then apply the split-thickness skin graft secondarily after edema has subsided.

In areas where the soft tissue envelope must be stress-competent or mobile relative to underlying layers, split-thickness skin should be applied as a temporary woundcover only.

Local Flaps

Advancement Flaps and Rotation Flaps. These classic techniques are used to resurface soft tissue defects of limited size occurring chiefly on the trunk, arm and thigh. They may be utilized only if the tissues surrounding the wound are not too severely crushed. In the lower leg, the bridge flap of Picot has achieved some importance in the primary closure of soft tissue defects over the anterior surface of the tibia. We cover the posterior donor site primarily with meshed split-thickness skin.

Muscle Flaps and Myocutaneous Flaps. These techniques may be performed also primarily. However, they are simple and safe when used for the secondary coverage of soft tissue defects of moderate size. With improved knowledge about the blood supply of specific muscles and the overlying skin, muscle flaps and myocutaneous flaps have added an important chapter to reconstructive plastic surgery, especially of the lower extremity. When performing these techniques, it is necessary to consider not only the blood supply of the muscle in question, but also the permissible range of the transfer. Below we shall point out a few of the many muscle and myocutaneous flaps that are available.

The laterally-based tensor fasciae latae flap makes it possible to resurface the upper and mid-thigh, even posteriorally, over a width of about 10 cm. The method is relatively safe (Fig. 1).

The vastus intermedius and lateralis flap is excellent for covering medial and lateral defects of the proximal and mid-thigh by virtue of its good vascular pedicle and width. However, the large bulk of the muscles limits the range of the transfer.

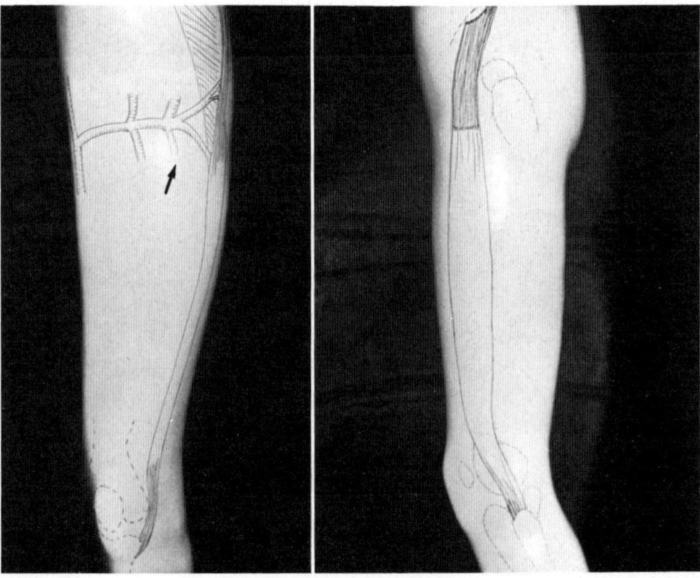

Fig. 1. Tensor fasciae latae flap based on the lateral femoral circumflex artery (*arrow*)

Owing to their length, the abductors are suitable for covering defects in the middle and distal thirds of the thigh, provided the defects are narrow. The extensor muscles of the thigh can in principle be used for myocutaneous flaps, but the resulting functional deficit limits the use of this group.

Muscle groups from the lower leg are available for covering defects about the knee. The proximally-based gastrocnemius muscles can provide good coverage of defects 15–18 cm long and 8–10 cm wide (Fig. 2). The three vascular pedicles of these muscles enable them to be mobilized from either the proximal or distal side, allowing defect coverage from the mid- to distal portion of the lower leg. Limited malleolar coverage can also be procured with special techniques. The medial gastrocnemius is used more frequently owing to its greater range.

The soleus is a broad, fan-shaped muscle with a good double or triple vascular pedicle, and as such is excellently suited for transpositions (Fig. 3). It can be used to cover large defects in the middle third of the lower leg and at the junction of the middle and distal thirds. Split-thickness skin is grafted onto the transposed muscle. The extensor hallucis longus and other muscles of the lower leg and foot (Fig. 4) may be used to cover defects of limited size. Details on these techniques may be found in the specialized literature.

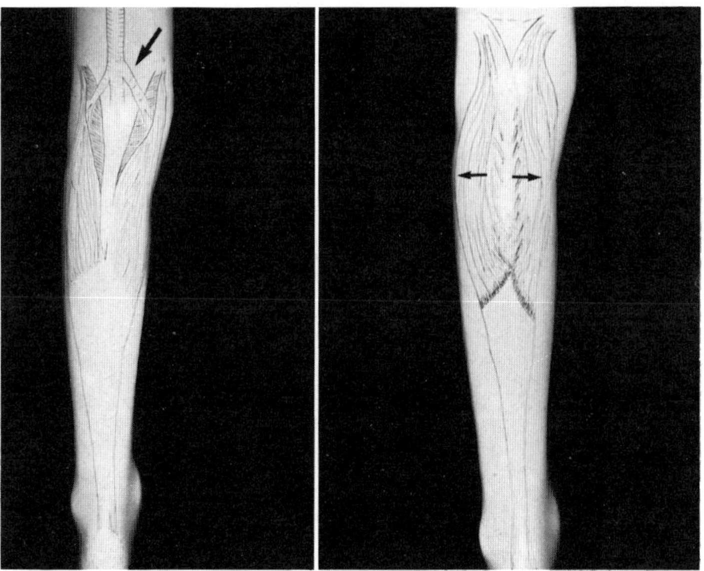

Fig. 2. Vascular pedicles of the gastrocnemius muscles. The *top arrow* points to the sural artery, and the *lower arrows* to its muscular ramii

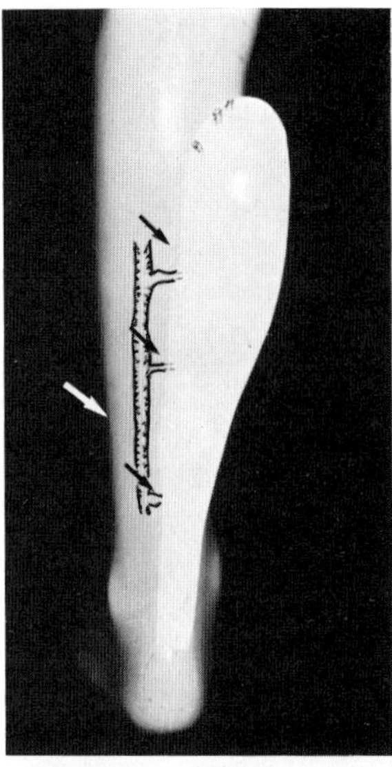

Fig. 3. The soleus muscle, schematically retracted to demonstrate its blood supply: The arrows mark the posterior tibial artery and its muscular ramii

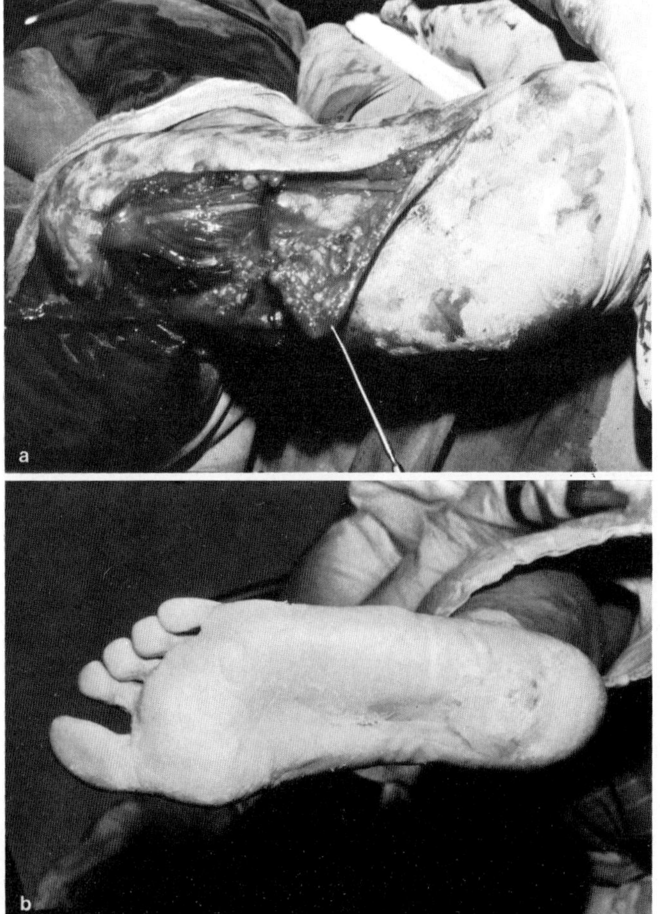

Fig. 4a, b. Open injury of the calcaneus in a 60-year-old man treated by muscle transposition (flexor digitorum brevis) and full-thickness skin grafting

Distant Flaps

Cross-leg Flaps. The cross-leg flap is the classic distant flap technique for the lower extremity. It enables even large defects to be covered with skin and subcutaneous tissue (Fig. 5). An important consideration with this method, however, is the impairment of joint mobility that may result from 3–4 weeks' immobilization of the legs.

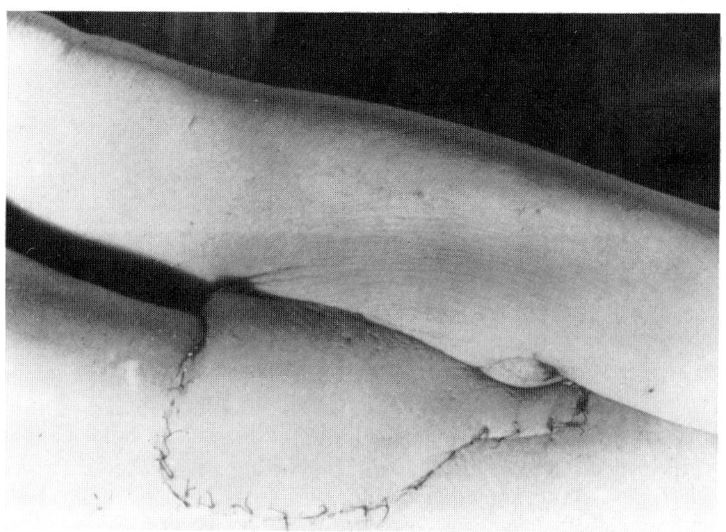

Fig. 5. "Classic" cross-leg flap from the posterior side of the right lower leg to the anterior side of the left lower leg. The donor site is covered primarily with split-thickness skin

Door Leave Flap. The door leave flap-technique is used to cover extensive defects on the anterior aspect of the lower leg. The operative technique will be briefly described:

After the traumatized soft tissues have been excised and the fracture stabilized, the lower leg on the uninjured side is approximated to the soft tissue defect so that the axial orientation of the proposed double flap transfer can be determined. The skin on the posterior side of the healthy lower leg is then incised down to the fascia, and a skin flap is dissected free on each side of the incision in door-leave-like fashion. The posterior incision may be straight, curved or even S-shaped, depending on the size and localization of the defect. Next the two extremities are apposed, and the edges of the elevated flaps are sutured to the edges of the defect. In this way the defect is covered not only by skin and subcutaneous tissue, but also by fascia. The relative position of the legs is maintained with an external fixator. Residual defects that cannot be covered with the flaps may be closed intraoperatively with split-thickness skin. Three to four weeks are allowed for incorporation of the flaps, after which time they are divided at the base in standard fashion, taking care not to separate the fascia from the bone or soft tissue of the injured leg. If the two flaps do not provide adequate coverage, a complete closure can still be obtained by grafting free skin onto the transplanted fascia. We have had much success with the door leave flap technique (Fig. 6). It is simple to perform, can be done primarily, and gives the experienced plastic surgeon a powerful tool for secondary reconstructions of the lower extremity.

Other distant flaps include the groin flap and the abdominal flap for soft tissue injuries of the hand and forearm. Flaps from the upper arm and forearm can be used to resurface defects on the contralateral hand. Flap thickness is an important consideration in this region.

Microvascular Free Flaps

The ability to anastomose vessels 1/2 mm or less in diameter through microsurgical techniques has greatly advanced the reconstructive surgery of severe soft tissue injuries. Developments in this area are rapid, and numerous potential donor sites have been described. This type of tissue transfer is rarely suitable as a primary measure. Of the fifty or so microvascular free flaps that are available, four will be described here:

Groin Flap. The groin flap, based on the superficial and/or deep circumflex iliac artery, is most important because of its length, which ranges to 20 cm. The flap is composed of skin and subcutaneous tissue. The main disadvantage of the flap is its short vascular pedicle, often making it necessary to interpose a vein graft in order to achieve a good anastomosis (especially in the extremities).

Tensor Fasciae Latae Flap. This free flap is used with increasing frequency. It possesses a good vascular pedicle up to 10 cm in length and, being composed of muscle, subcutaneous tissue and skin, provides an even better material for the coverage and reconstruction of large soft tissue defects. By preserving the nerve supply to the flap, it is possible to retain some degree of muscular function.

Latissimus Dorsi Flap. This flap is the most widely used at the present time. Its pedicle, consisting of the thoracodorsal artery and vein, can be mobilized over a length of 12 cm or more. This circumstance, plus the presence of the thoracodorsal nerve, enables the transplantation of a functioning muscular unit. A further advantage of the latissimus dorsi flap is the relative ease of primary closure of the donor site. The flap may be up to 28 cm long and 18 cm wide, in which case the donor site is resurfaced with split-thickness skin. A disadvantage of the technique is the necessity of transfering a very thick muscle mass.

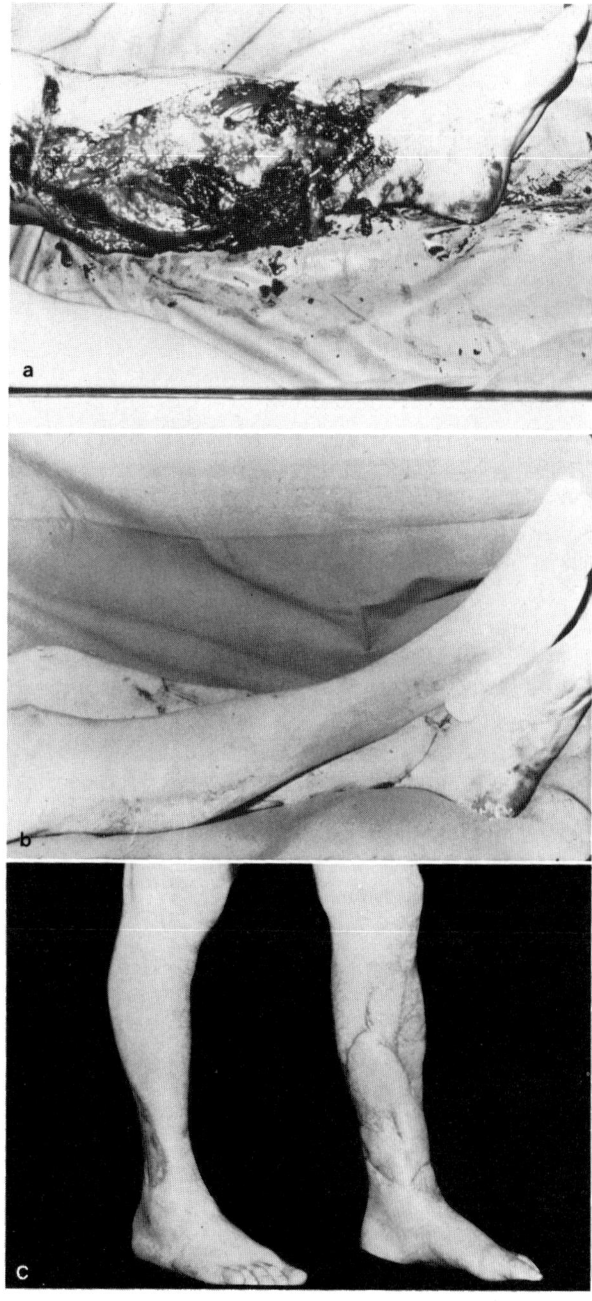

Fig. 6. a Severe open fracture of the left tibia in a 50-year-old man. **b** The defect was covered primarily with door leave flap from the right lower leg, with split-thickness skin grafts used to cover residual defects. **c** The functional result at 3 years is very good.

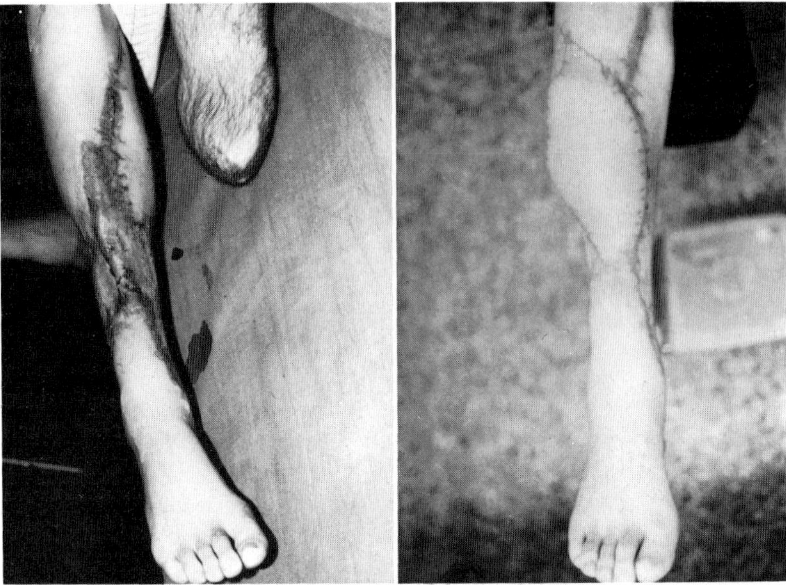

Fig. 7. Open fracture of the right tibia and below-knee amputation of the left leg in a male aged 17 years. The defect was covered initially with a meshed split-thickness skin graft. A free latissimus dorsi flap with neuroanastomosis was performed secondarily

The possibility of using the latissimus dorsi flap as a functioning muscular unit to replace other muscle groups is illustrated by the case in Fig. 7. In this patient the nerve of latissimus dorsi was anastomosed to the fibular nerve at the time of the transfer. Five months later the muscle showed significant contraction and was able to assist in gait.

If atrophy of the oversize muscle belly is desired, this may be induced by dispensing with the neuroanastomosis. In this case the muscle functions simply as a mediator of blood flow to the transplanted skin. In time the muscle will become atrophied and fibrotic.

The latissimus dorsi flap can also be used as an island flap for repairing circumscribed defects of the lower leg. This flap contains only that portion of the muscle which directly underlies the transplanted skin, and selective dissection of the nutrient vessels is required (Fig. 8). The latissimus tendon and the bulk of the muscle mass are not used.

Neurovascular Dorsalis Pedis Flap. This flap provides skin and subcutaneous tissue coverage of defects up to 10 x 8 cm in size and is used mainly on the hand. Sensation can also be restored by anastomosing nerve branches in the flap to recipient nerves at the host site.

A new and useful flap, which should be mentioned is the radial artery neurovascular flap.

Mention should also be made of the capabilities offered by compositve microvascular tissue transfers in the reconstruction of cutaneous, subcutaneous, muscular and osseous defects. The fibula, ilium and ribs are the major sources of osteocutaneous grafts for these procedures.

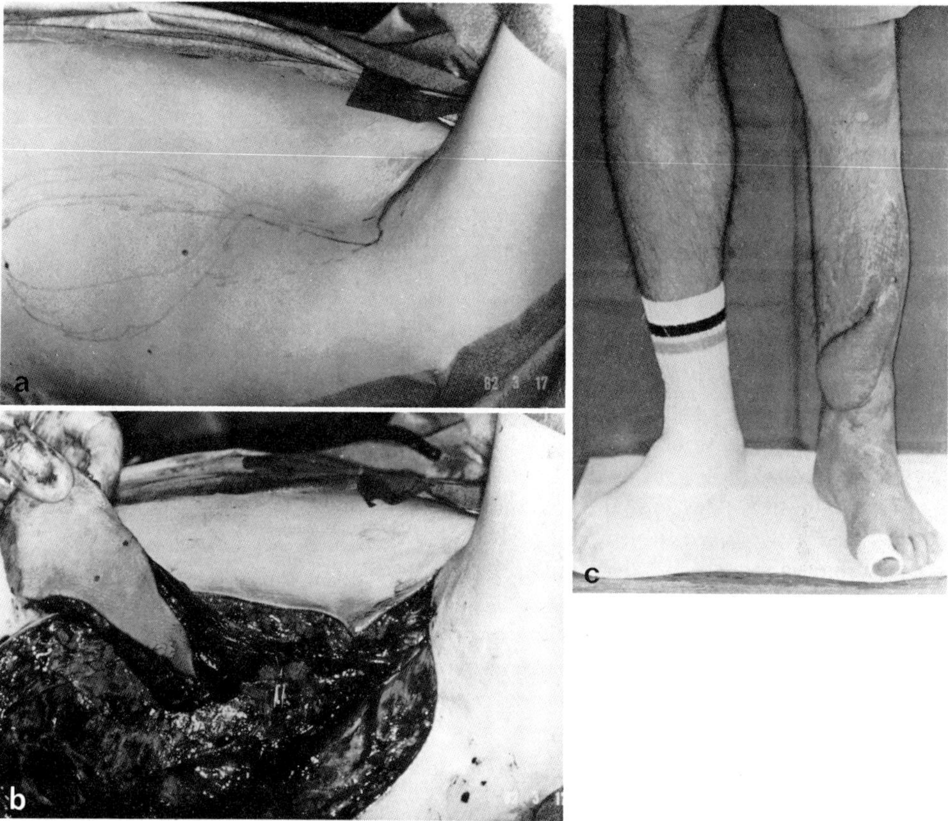

Fig. 8a–c. Latissimus dorsi flap with a long muscular and vascular pedicle, mobilized as an island flap containing a narrow strip of skin (**a**, **b**) and used to resurface the left lower leg following an open comminuted fracture (**c**)

Finally, with regard to the technique of the free tissue transfers, it should be emphasized that a detailed angiographic examination of the blood vessels of both the donor and recipient sites is an absolute prerequisite before surgery is done.

2. Conclusions

The successful treatment of severe soft tissue lesions, which often are associated with osseous injuries, must be based upon a clear conceptual approach in which primary and secondary care constitute a unit.

Primary Care

The main components of primary care are:

- Meticulous wound debridement.
- Stable operative fixation of the fracture.
- Primary coverage of soft tissue defects. This is usually done with a synthetic skin dressing, but split-thickness skin grafts may be applied to a healthy wound bed, and local or distant flaps may be used in some instances.

Secondary Plastic Reconstruction

The definitive closure of the defect and the reconstruction of damaged functional units represent a continuation of primary care and should not be deferred for more than a few days. The selection of a technique from among the many flap advancements, muscle transpositions, free flaps and free tissue transfers available is governd by local circumstances. The experienced surgeon will choose the specific plastic surgical technique that is more promising in terms of the ultimate functional result.

References

1. Berger A, Meissl G, Piza H (1975) Free flap in emergency surgery. Proc. Europ Congr of Emerg Surg, Paris
2. Brück HG (1961) Zur Verwendung des sogenannten Cross-leg-flap. Seine Indikationen und Kontraindikationen. Langenbecks Arch Chir 299:156
3. McCraw JB, Dibbell DG, Carraway JH (1977) Experimental definition of independent myocutaneous vascular territories. Plast Reconstr Surg 60:212
4. Ger R (1976) The coverage of vascular repairs by muscle transposition. J Trauma 16: 974
5. McGregor IA, Jackson IA (1972) The groin flap. Brit J Plast Surg 25:3
6. Marii K, Ohmori K, Sekiguchi J (1976) The free muscle musculotaneous flap. Plast Reconstr Surg 57:294
7. Kutscha-Lissberg E, Meiss G, Millesi H, Trojan E (1975) Erfahrungen mit der erweiterten Lappenplastik zur primären Deckung großer Hautdefekte bei offenen Unterschenkelbrüchen. Chir Praxis 20:91
8. Millesi H, Trojan E (1969) Zur primären Lappenplastik bei schweren offenen Unterschenkelbrüchen. Akt Chir Austr 3:49
9. Millesi H, Spängler HP (1966) Zur Behandlung infizierter Knochenwunden durch gestielte Hauttransplantation. Münch med Wschr 108:2193
10. Orticochea M (1972) The musculotaneous flap method. Brit Plast Surg 25:106
11. Stangl Th, Vaubel E, Enes-Gaiao F (1981) Indikation und Technik des myocutanen Cross-leg-Lappens. Hefte Unfallheilkd
12. Taylor GI, Daniel RK (1973) The free flap: composite tissue-transfer by vascular anastomosis. Aust N Z J Surg 43:1
13. Vogt B (1963) Zur Technik der Überkreuzplastik. Chirurg 34:326

Replantation Surgery: Indications and Limitations

A. Berger

1. Introduction

The ability to successfully repair minute structures under the operating microscope was first utilized in replantation surgery, and in fact accounts for the high success rate and widespread use of the procedure. Since the establishment of replantation centers in Central Europe, the first of which was instituted in Vienna in 1974, experience with the procedure has become available in a large number of patients. Moreover, based on an evaluation of longer-term results, it is now possible to set forth the indications for surgical replantation in fairly specific terms.

The success or failure of replantation surgery, including both micro- and macroreplantations, depends upon four factors:

a) Recognition and initial evaluation of the injury and the organization of transport.
b) Availability of an in-hospital replantation service and notification of the replantation team.
c) Level of equipment, technique and training of the attending microsurgeons.
d) Sound postoperative management.

A review of the numberous replantations performed during my years in Vienna and more recently in Hannover demonstrates the indications and limitations of the procedure, which have met with international acceptance.

2. Injury Classification and Clinical Material

The injuries may be classified into three groups according to severity:

1. complete amputations,
2. incomplete amputations,
3. injuries in which basic blood flow is preserved.

Complete amputations are clearly defined. Incomplete amputations take various forms and may be subdivided into five groups. In all cases, however, the injured part would be unable to survive without restoration of its blood supply.

In injuries of the third group, disruption of the blood supply is partial, and an effort is made to restore the initial blood flow.

Our clinical material comprises 628 cases from the Viennese Replantation Center and 400 cases treated in Hannover Medical School. 82 amputated parts from 298 of the Vienna patients and 252 amputated parts from 162 of the Hannover patients were replanted using microsurgical technique. Thirty-eight percent were guillotine injuries, 21% mild crush, 20% severe crush, 12% avulsions, and 9% degloving injuries (Table 1). The patients ranged in age from 18 months to 71 years.

Table 1. Types of injury

Guillotine injury	38%
Mild crush	21%
Severe crush	20%
Avulsion	12%
Degloving	9%

The third group, in which a basic circulation was still present, is excluded from the present review.

3. Emergency Care and Transport

The most important aspect of emergency care are recognition of the injury, preservation of the amputated part, and hemostasis, all without inflicting additional trauma. A completely amputated part should be cooled to a temperature no lower than 4°C. Under no circumstances should it be frozen. The safest method is to seal the part in a plastic bag, placing this in a second plastic bag containing ice cubes and water. The amputated part should not come in contact with the ice or water (Fig. 1).

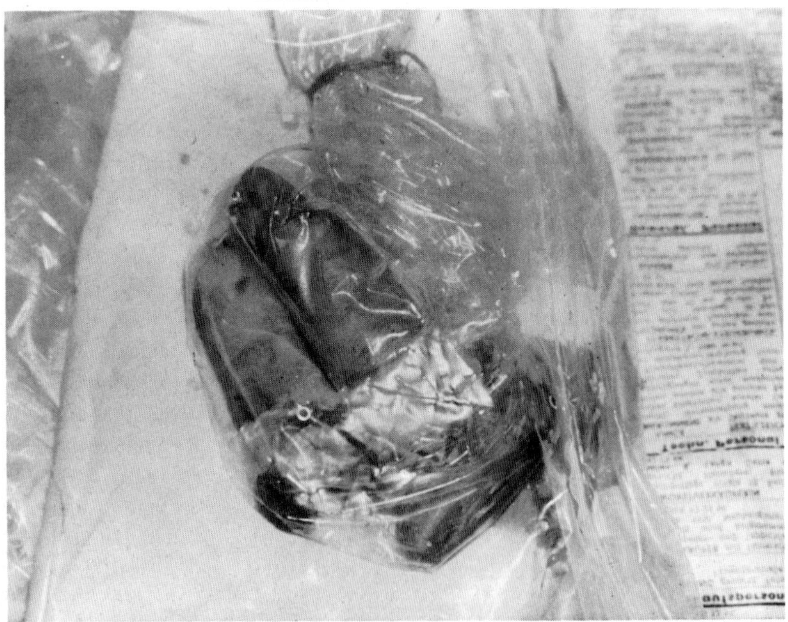

Fig. 1. The amputated part is sealed in a double plastic bag with ice cubes and water between the walls of the bags

With an incomplete amputation, cooling is not indicated, but the involved joints should be splinted in an intermediate position, with care taken to reappose structures in their approximate anatomical positions.

Four hours' warm ischemia or 8–10 hours' cold ischemia is acceptable in minor replantations.

In major replantations, a warm ischemic time of 2–4 hours or cold ischemic time of 6 hours is still considered acceptable. This ischemic time must include operating time, i.e., the time until arterial anastomosis is established.

Thus, notification of the replantation unit is an essential phase of emergency care, for these procedures not only require specialized equipment and instrumentation, but also tie up the operating room for long periods of time.

4. Organization of an In-Hospital Replantation Service

By international agreement, replantation facilities are categorized according to the level of service which they provide. In replantation centers, a replantation team is available on a 24-hour basis, enabling replantations to be performed on demand. A replantation service of this type is available at Hannover Medical School. There are other hospitals in which replantations are performed, but only within the framework of normal services.

An important factor in the organization of an in-hospital replantation service are facilities for training members of the replantation team in an experimental microsurgical program.

5. Operative Technique

The technique of replantation surgery, and especially replantation microsurgery, has become so standardized that predictable results generally can be achieved for a given degree of injury. The use of small micro-vein grafts in particular has done much to broaden the range of replantation surgery.

Preparation should begin on the stump, as the vascular pedicle is identified and its suitability for anastomosis is evaluated. The amputated part is then examined to assess the quality of its vessels and determine whether its overall condition is suitable for replantation (secondary injuries). Cooling of the part is maintained during this time.

If the decision favors replantation, it is necessary first to shorten the bone as a prelude to achieving good soft tissue closure. Bone shortening prior to internal fixation is done solely for that purpose and not, as once believed, to permit a tension-free anastomosis of the vessels. Residual defects between vascular stumps are bridged with interposition vein grafts.

The next step is to stabilize the fracture, using plates and screws on the metacarpals and more proximal bones (Fig. 2), and Kirschner wires on the digits. It is essential that adequate stability be achieved when the latter method is used.

For injuries involving the proximal or distal interphalangeal joint, a primary arthrodesis should be performed if reconstruction of the joint is not feasible.

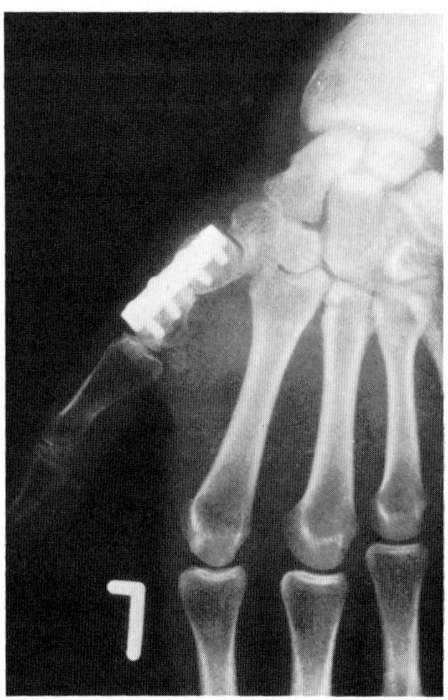

Fig. 2. Plate fixation of the 1st metacarpal

After the bony injuries have been dealt with, repairs are carried out on the extensor tendon and extensor aponeurosis. The flexor tendons are anastomosed by the method of Kleinert. Next the palmar digital nerves are repaired if possible, especially on the radial side. If damage is too severe, grafting may be done later as a secondary procedure. Nerve repair is followed by restoration of the arterial flow. At least one artery should be repaired, and two arteries are preferable to one. If the slightest tension occurs, vein grafts taken from the forearm or forefoot should be interposed. Ideally, twice as many veins as arteries should be available for venous outflow. However, one large vein may be sufficient if the remaining veins are ligated so that the main flow is diverted to that vein.

As soon as the clamps are released and arterial flow is reestablished, the infusion of low molecular weight dextran is begun. When the operation is complete and the circulatory status of the replanted part is judged to be satisfactory, a plaster cast is applied over ample padding. Joints should be in a functional position when the cast is applied. Postoperative elevation of the extremity between 30° and 45° has proved beneficial. Over the next 4–5 days, low molecular weight dextran is administered in a dose of 250 ml twice daily, and vasodilators and antithrombotic agents are also administered during this time. Antibiotics are indicated for heavily contaminated wounds.

6. Postoperative Care and Rehabilitation

A sound program of postoperative physical and occupational therapy is an integral part of the total treatment plan. It is especially important that the patient be well motivated during this phase. Appropriate rehabilitation measures reinforced by personal guidance for each individual patient can produce astonishing functional results even if the replantation was not technically perfect. It is imperative that physical therapy be continued for a sufficiently long period and, if possible, administered intermittently under inpatient conditions.

7. Secondary Procedures

Secondary procedures were undertaken in 40% of the patients in our review. They were done mainly for the purpose of improving function and consisted largely of tendon and nerve reconstructions and corrections of malunions. Disturbances of fracture healing were another frequent indication for secondary surgery. Osteitis or pseudarthroses was present in 15% of cases. Only 3% of the patients required reamputation.

8. Follow-Ups

Sixty-five patients who had undergone replantation surgery were reexamined after a minimum of two years, and the results were assessed both objectively and subjectively. All of these replantations had been performed distal to the wrist. The replantation of 11 upper extremities and 5 forearms were reviewed separately.

The hand and digital replantations were evaluated objectively by means of function tests administered by someone other than the attending physician: two-point discrimination, force of power grip and pinch (measured in bar), temperature adaptation, and range of individual finger motion.

Table 2 shows that the power grip of the replanted thumb was good compared to the healthy side. The difference relative to the healthy side was minimal, averaging 0.11 bar. Two-point discrimination ranged between 4 and 10 mm, with an average of 6 mm. Temperature adaption was of good quality. Key pinch and tip-to-tip pinch were positive in 80% of cases.

As Table 3 shows, the replanted index finger also had a power grip comparable to that of the uninjured side. Two-point discrimination was 8 mm on the average, and temperature adaption was 50%.

The results for the middle and ring fingers were similar but generally poorer (Table 4).

The subjective assessment of the results was based upon the degree of "integration" of the replanted part into daily and occupational activities. We found that full integration had taken place in 53% of the patients (Table 5). Twenty-five percent had to have retraining before a full integration could be achieved. This means that 78% of the patients profitted from their replantation.

In 12% the replanted part could not be integrated into normal activities without significant disability, but none of these patients expressed a desire for reamputation. In 5% the replanted part significantly hampered the overall function of the hand. Another 5% could not be evaluated.

The results of upper-extremity and forearm replantations were rated much more favorably by the patients than by the examiner. The patients were pleased to have retained an arm which, despite significant functional disability, nevertheless had sensation and could

Table 2. Functional results in replanted thumbs

Patient		Power grip in bar	Temperature 0–2	2 PD (mm)	Opposition	Flexion	Key pinch	Tip-to-tip pinch
25	(I)	0.10–0.38	2	6	reduced	–	+	+/2nd finger
72	(I)	0.21–0.25	2	4	normal	+	+	+
49	(I)	0.50–0.42	1	8	normal	++	+	+
70	(I)	0.20–0.32	1	10/Prot.	normal	–	+	+
69	(I)	0.15–0.50	1–2	8	normal	+ –	+	+
48	(I)	0.15–0.20	0–1	10	normal	reduced	+	+
82	(I)	0.08–0.20	2	8	normal	reduced	+	+
39	(M)	0.09–0.13	1–2	10	reduced	+ –	+ –	+
66	(M)	0.17–0.28	2	–/Prot.	normal	+	+ –	+
1	(M) left	0.05–0.45	0–1	6–10	severely reduced	reduced	+ – (1–2)	– (1–2)
1	(M) right	0.15	2	10		–	+ – (1–3)	– (1–3)
27	(M)	0.18–0.20	2	6	normal	reduced	+	+ –

Table 3. Functional results in replanted index fingers

Patient		Power grip (bar)	Temperature adaption 0–2	2 PD (mm)	FTPD (cm)
52	(I)	0.15–0.86	0	0	6
43	(I)	0.18–0.48	2	10	2.5
2	(I)	0.20	2	10	9
56	(I)	0.00	1	10	0
92	(I)	0.45	2	3	0
12	(I)	0.11–0.29	2	3	0.8
51	(I)	0.32	2	4–6	5
10	(M)	0.10–0.34	1–2	10	8
44	(M)	0.43	2	6–10	5
80	(M)	0.20–0.35	1	0	3.5
68	(M)	0.15–0.20	2	6	4
39	(M)	0.09–0.26	2	10	9
1	(M)	0	2	8	5
27	(M)	0.2	1	Prot.	3.5

Table 4. Functional results in replanted middle and ring fingers

Middle finger

Patient		Power grip (bar)	Temperature adaption 0–2	2 PD (mm)	FTPD (cm)
29	(I)	0.30–0.90	2	2–4	0
44	(M)	0.43	1	5	8
10	(M)	0.30	0	10	4
80	(M)	0.20–0.35	1	0	2.5
68	(M)	0.15	2	6	8
1	(M)	–	2	4	9

Ring finger

Patient		Power grip (bar)	Temperature adaptation 0–2	2 PD (mm)	FTPD (cm)
18	(I)	0.58	2	4	0
13	(I)	0.17–0.9	2	6	0
64	(I)	0.12	2	0	0
66	(M)	0.66	2	3	7
68	(M)	–	2	4	0

Table 5. Functional result – Integration

Replanted part	Integrated	53%	78%
	Retrained	25%	
Replanted part not integrated		12%	
Replanted part hampers overall function		5%	
Not evaluated		5%	

Table 6. Macroremplantations

Upper extremity			Forearm	
11 (4)			5	(2)
Replanted	9	(4)	5	(2)
Reamputated	5	(2)	0	
Mortality	2	(0)	0	
Success	4	(2)	5	(2)

(Hannover patients enclosed in parentheses.)

be used to assist the healthy extremity. They prefer this state over an insensible prosthesis (Table 6).

When questioned, all the patients stated that they would undergo the replantation again. The age of the patients had no influence on the replantation itself or the usefulness of the replanted parts.

9. Rheographic and Thermometric Follow-Ups

Follow-up blood flow measurements were carried out in 24% of the replantations for complete amputations, as well as in 38 partially-amputated digits. Even two or three years after replantation, longitudinal rheography showed typical changes such as a disturbance of venous return or patterns characteristic of sympathetic blockade. The rheographic quotient of complete amputations showed that the blood flow in the replanted part was still markedly decreased relative to the healthy side. In incomplete amputations this discrepancy was less pronounced.

Functional extremital thermometry, used to assess the capacity of the injured part for adaptation to temperature changes, showed little difference between the injured and uninjured sides in cases where the replanted part was revascularized and had good nerve regeneration. In cases of complete amputation, however, marked differences in response to cold stimuli persisted even after two years. This was also documented by gradual rewarming of the part after cooling to 15°.

It would appear, then, that intact vasomotor fibers have a critical bearing on the quality of the end result. We are investigating this problem more closely in a new study.

10. Remarks on Patient Selection

The current criteria for the selection of replantation candidates may be summarized as follows:

Replantation is definitely indicated in:

- Amputations of the thumb (Figs. 3, 4)
- Amputations of more than one finger (Fig. 5)
- Amputations of the hand (Fig. 6)
- Pediatric patients.

Replantation may be indicated in:

- Amputations of a single finger. The decision is influenced by the patient's occupation, hobbies and wishes. Informed consent is essential.
- Amputations of the lower extremity, if satisfactory results can be expected from a well-fitting prosthesis.

The nature of the injury is another factor to be considered when selecting candidates for replantation. The best results are achieved in sharp amputations or mild crush amputations without massive tissue trauma. Avulsions and degloving injuries carry a poorer prognosis.

Replantation is not feasible when there is massive damage to the amputated part or stump, or in patients with severe or life-threatening associated injuries. The final decision should rest with a physician who is experienced in microsurgery and surgery of the hand.

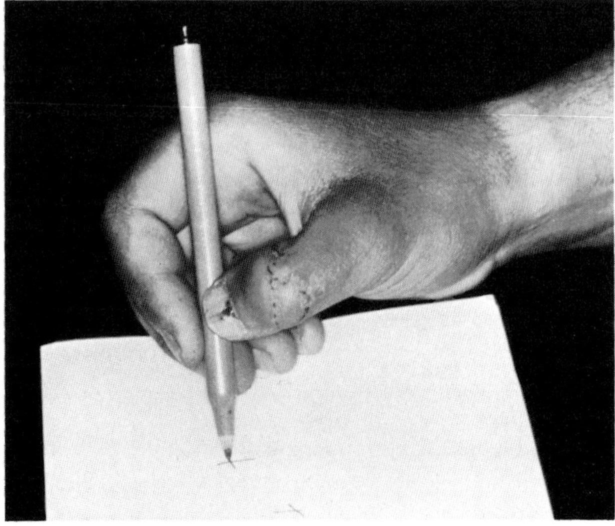

Fig. 3. 30-year-old man with a replanted right thumb that had been completely amputated through its midportion; function three years later

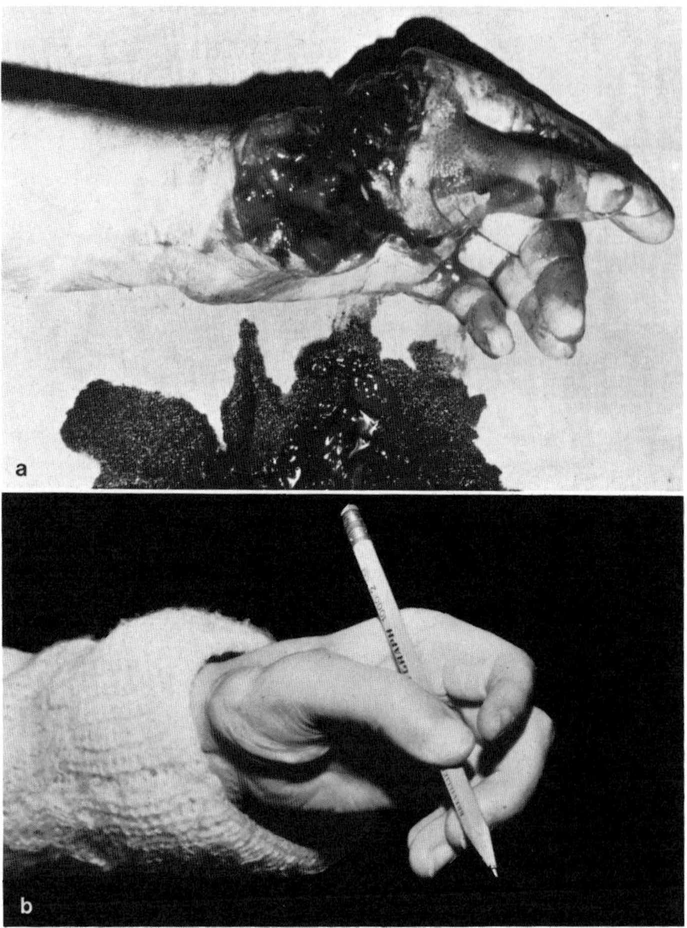

Fig. 4. a Complete amputation of the thumb and incomplete amputation of the index finger of the left hand in a 20-year-old female. **b** Good functional result two years later

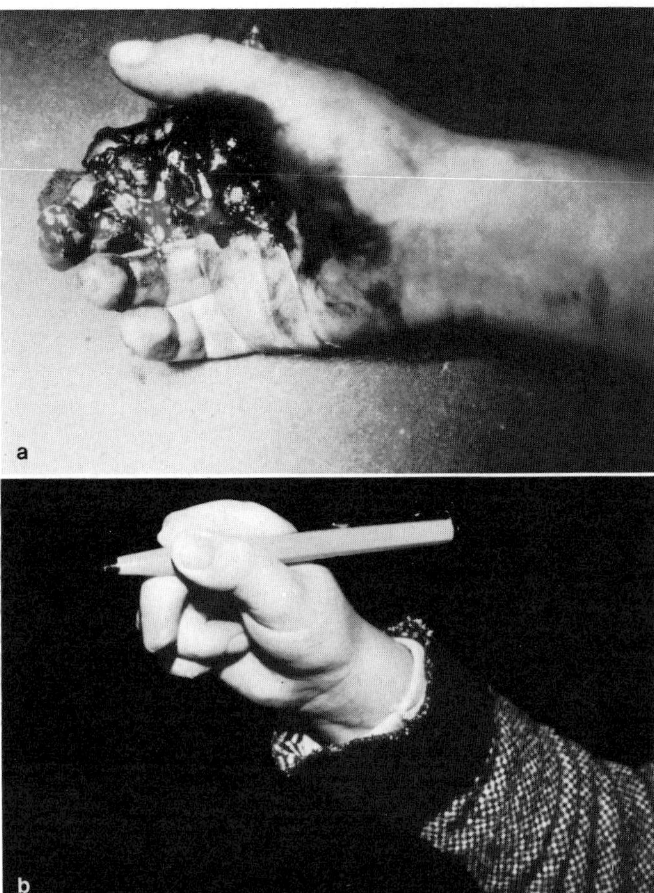

Fig. 5. a Complete amputation of the 2nd finger and incomplete amputation of the 3rd finger of the right hand in an 8-year-old boy. **b** Functional result one year after replantation

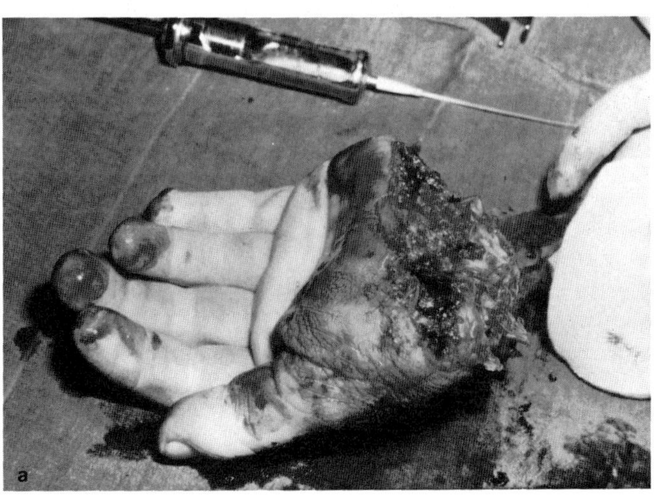

Fig. 6. Punch injury with complete amputation of both hands in a male aged 17 years. **a** Left hand

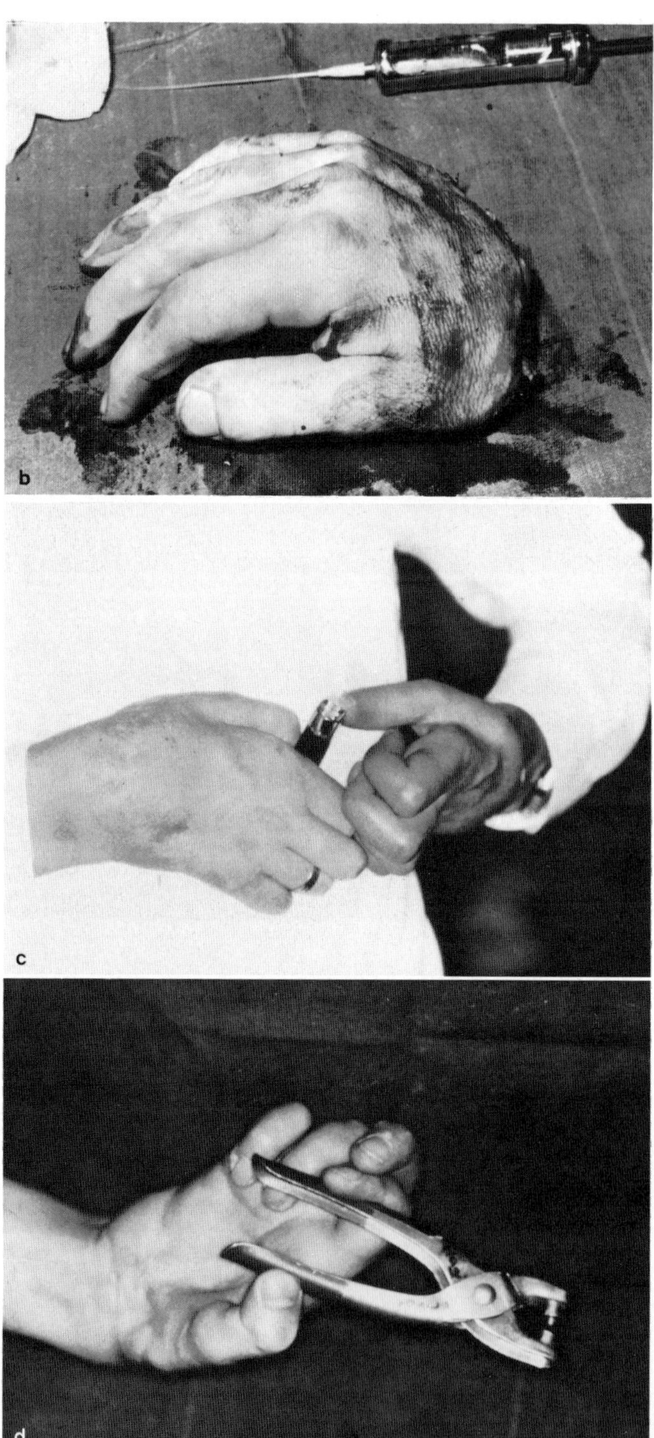

Fig. 6. Punch injury with complete amputation of both hands in a male aged 17 years. **b** Right hand. **c, d** Three years later the replanted parts are completely integrated into daily and occupational activities

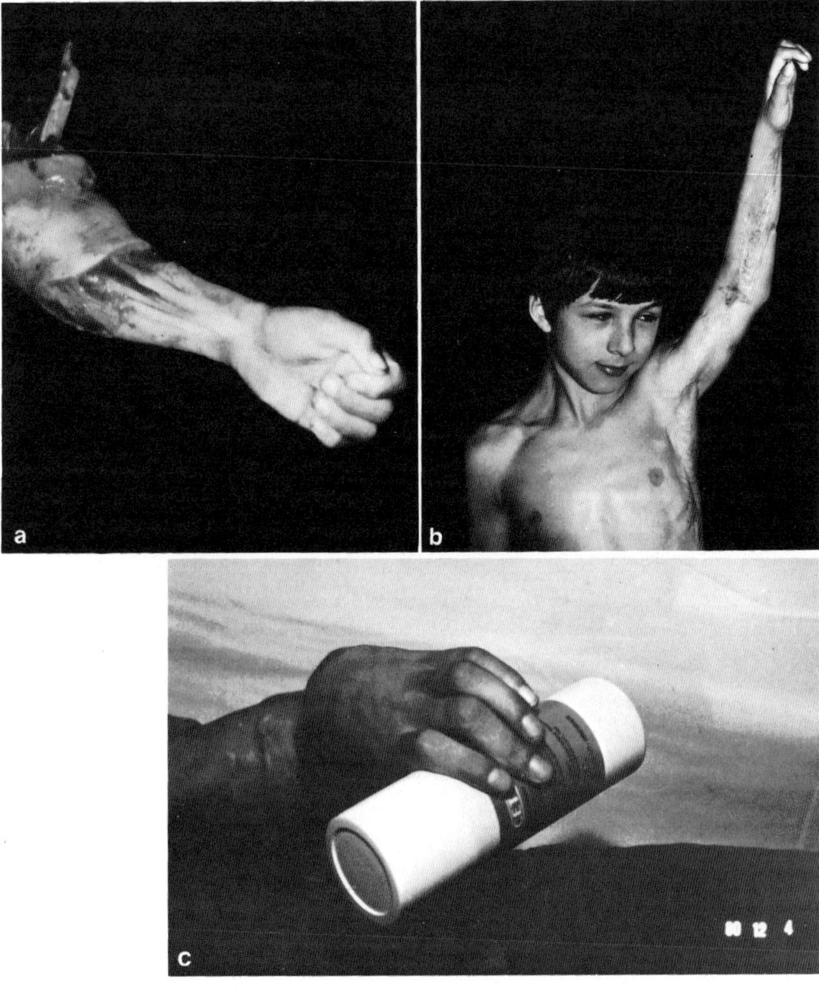

Fig. 7a–c. Loss of the left arm with severe traumatization of the forearm in a 9-year-old boy (**a**). Appearance four years after replantation (**b**) and functional result (**c**)

11. Concluding Remarks

Replantation surgery can no longer be considered to be in its initial stages, and its indications and limits are clear. Previous experience and an objective appraisal of follow-up results shows replantation surgery to be an effective branch of plastic and rehabilitation surgery of the members, and it can make a significant contribution in reducing the consequences of severe injuries to the extremities. It requires, however, specially trained surgeons practising in large centers who are in command of the entire spectrum of appropriate methods of treatment and who are constantly available to perform operations. Only in this way can the high standard that has thus far been maintained continue and be improved upon.

References

1. Alperts BS, Buncke HJ, Brownstein M (1978) Replacement of damaged arteries and veins with vein grafts when replanting crushed, amputated fingers. Plast Reconstr Surg 30:17
2. Anderl H, Hussl H, Bauer M, Martin R, Riege W, Papp Ch (1979) Die Replantation von Fingern und Gliedmaßen. Akt Traumatol 9:223
3. Berger A, Meissl G, Millesi H, Piza H, Walzer L, Mandl H, Frey G (1978) Replantation of extremities – experiences of the Viennese replantation team after four years of work. Excerpta Med, Int Congr 465, Mikrosurg
4. Berger A, Millesi H (1980) Functional results in replantation surgery, five years experience of the Viennese replantation team. Aust New Zealand Journ Surg 3:122
5. Berger A, Meisl G, Millesi H, Walzer L (1980) Vein grafts in microvascular surgery of the hand. First congress of the International Societies for Surgery of the Hand, Rotterdam
6. Berger A, Brühne B, Walzer R (1979) Functional tests in the follow up of study of replanted tissues and hands. Proc Int Congr of Plast Surg, Rio de Janeiro
7. Berger A (1981) Spezielle Indikation in der mikrochirurgischen Unfallchirurgie – Daumenreplantation. Hefte Unfallheilkd 162
8. Berger H (1981) Organization of a replantation service – seven years of experiences. 29. Congr d Societe Int d Chir, Montreux
9. Biemer E (1979) Vein grafts in microvascular surgery. Br J Plast Surg 30:197
10. Biemer E (1981) Daumenersatztechnik. Hefte Unfallheilkd
11. O'Brien B (1977) Microvascular reconstructive surgery. Churchill Livingstone, Edinburgh
12. Buck-Gramcko D (1978) Funktionelle Spätergebnisse der mikrovaskulären Chirurgie. Handchir 10:81
13. Cobbett JR (1969) Free digital transfer. J Bone Joint Surg 51:677
14. Duspiva W, Biemer E, Hanfmann B (1981) Zur Indikation der Replantation einzelner Finger. Hefte Unfallheilkd
15. Jacobson JH, Suarez EL (1960) Microsurgery in the anastomoses of small vessels. Surg Forum 11:243
16. Klammer HL, Schulz RF (1981) Langzeitergebnisse und sozialökonomische Effizienz bei Makroreplantationen. Hefte Unfallheilkd
17. Owen E (1975) Replantation of amputated extremities. Langenbecks Arch Chir 339: 613
18. Pennig D, Brug E (1981) Die prognostische Bedeutung der muskulären pH-Registrierung in der Replantationschirurgie. Hefte Unfallheilkd
19. Tamai S (1974) Present status and prospect of limb and finger replantation. Surg Diag Treat 6:547
20. Wayne A, Morrison B, O'Brien BM, MacLeod AM (1979) Evaluation of digital replantation – a review of 100 cases. Orthop N Am 8:2
21. Zwank L, Schweiberer L, Hertel P (1978) Indikation, Technik und Ergebnisse bei Klein- und Großreplantationen. Plast Chir 2:133

Subject Index